FOOD IS
Medicine

101 PRESCRIPTIONS
FROM THE GARDEN

KATHLEEN BARNES

TAKE
CHARGE
BOOKS

Brevard, North Carolina

Contains material adapted and abridged from *Rx From the Garden* by Kathleen Barnes. Copyright © 2011 by F+W Media, Inc. Reprinted with permission. All Rights Reserved.

Library of Congress Cataloging-in-Publication Data is on file with the Library of Congress.

ISBN: 978-0-99615-890-9

Typesetting and cover design: Gary A. Rosenberg
Editor: Kathleen Barnes

Printed in the United States of America

10   9   8   7   6   5   4   3   2   1

Contents

PART 3 Superfoods You Can Grow, 137

Introduction

There is a certain romance to growing your own food. Whether it comes from a solitary basil plant on a window ledge, a potted tomato on an urban balcony, a small plot in a community garden or a well-manicured full-scale spread, we humans take pride in growing our own food, feeding ourselves and relishing the flavor and vitality our home grown foods bring to our bodies and spirits.

Most of us are aware that eating five or more servings of fruits and vegetables daily can prevent and even treat a host of diseases and illnesses. More and more of us are becoming aware of the importance of eating fresh wholesome local food that can keep us healthy, prevent disease and extend our lives. Many of us are trying to save money by growing our own food. Some of us even know the secrets of treating ailments and illnesses with herbs, fruits and vegetables.

In this book, I hope to make those secrets common knowledge. I'm here to share with you the road to good health through the freshest of fruits and vegetables. I'll share with you what I've learned about health and healing with the right foods grown the right way. I'll share with you some of my successes, failures and insights gained from a lifetime of gardening. I don't expect that you can or will grow every fruit and vegetable mentioned in this book. Most of us simply don't have the time or space. But I promise to offer you the secrets of healing with everyday foods available to everyone close to home.

Back in the early '70s when I was just out of college, my friends and family thought I was a little wacky when I started talking about natural healing. They asked:

- Why brew a cup of sage tea when it was easier to take a swig of sugar-laden cough medicine?

- Why wrap an infected cut with chewed wood sorrel rather than slapping on a little triple antibiotic from a tube?

- Why chew a few fennel seeds or drink a cup of peppermint tea rather than take a Tums?

- Why compost my kitchen scraps when it is so easy to buy a bag of compost at the big-box garden center?

- Why slave away under a hot sun, watering and weeding and battling bugs and blights, when a juicy tomato was as close as my local supermarket?

Why? Because all of these remedies and a simple lifestyle contribute to health and longevity. Even when I was in my twenties, healthy and longevity were my goals. More than forty years later, they still are.

I've gardened all of my life. My earliest memories are of helping my grandmother weed her garden and gathering perfect roses wet with the morning dew. I've survived short growing seasons and harsh winters in northern New York State near the Canadian border. I've gardened in Asia and Africa, weathering the scorn of locals for my pitiful and often unsuccessful efforts.

Now I live in the mountains of western North Carolina, my gardens sprawl all over our one-acre property. They're not always neat; in fact, they're not often neat. My compost bins are as far from scientific as you can get; nevertheless, I get "black gold" with the help of Mother Nature and Father Time. I have my share of garden failures, sometimes due to environmental conditions beyond my control, more often due to my own shortcomings. And while I don't grow every morsel on our plates, in the summer I grow most of our vegetables and some of our fruit. I buy local whenever I can to support local growers and prevent the pollution associated with huge semis trucking produce across the country to my local supermarket.

In return, my garden has rewarded me with delicious food, good health, exercise that I enjoy, and a golden farmer's tan. My aim in this book is to help you reap the same rewards.

—Kathleen Barnes
Brevard, NC, February 2015

PART 1

Let Food Be
Your Medicine

There's nothing like biting into a juicy tomato, still warm from the summer sun. Many times, I am content to eat my entire meal right there in the garden. I can snap off an asparagus stalk or eat a tomato without even washing it because I don't use pesticides or herbicides in my garden.

We live on a gravel road a mile from the nearest highway. The two cars that pass by daily don't worry me in terms of adding hydrocarbons to my crops, but it's certainly something to think about if you garden in a city or near a busy highway.

We have a deep well so we are free of worry about additives to municipal water, and because we're at the top of a mountain very far from any agricultural enterprises, we're confident that our water quality is as good as it gets. In all, I think we avoid adding to our toxic load just about as much as is possible in modern society. We're not purists, but it's a pretty idyllic life, if you love mountains and fresh air and lots of space.

For many years, my husband and I lived in some of the world's biggest cities, but when the time came that, thanks to advancing technology, we could pursue our livelihoods almost anywhere, we high-tailed it to the Blue Ridge mountains of western North Carolina. We've never looked back. Our lifestyle isn't for everyone, but I hope one or two of my thoughts here will inspire you to make even the smallest baby steps toward a more independent and healthy food supply, no matter where you live.

If you're like-minded, please join me at www.kathleen barnes.com.

GROWING VS. BUYING LOCAL

It's nearly impossible to grow everything you eat. But beyond what you're able to grow, one of the best things you can do for your health and the health of the planet is to buy produce (and meat) as locally as possible. There are three major reasons why:

1. Locally grown food is fresher than anything that has been trucked in and therefore has more nutrients. Most foods begin to lose their nutrients the moment they are picked, so a tomato that grew in your backyard or in a garden three miles from you will have much more vitamin C, lycopene, beta-carotene, and other nutrients than one that traveled from California or Argentina.

   The veggies I don't grow come mostly from the farmer's market or the produce stand down the highway. I've quizzed the local growers about their methods. They're not officially organic, since organic certification is a long and complicated process, but I choose the ones that don't use pesticides or herbicides or GMO seeds. The local producers and most local farmers are as wary of GMO foods as I am, so the luscious sweet corn we get all summer comes from GMO-free fields.

   You probably have a farmer's market in your town—

even the smallest burgs and the biggest cities have them. Patronize your local farmers for your own health and to help boost your local economy.

2. The environmental cost of locally produced food is lower because we're not using gas to transport the food long distances. There's a concept called "food miles," which translates to "how much does your food really cost the environment when your lettuce is being trucked in from California to North Carolina?" Of course, what immediately follows is that a $3 plastic carton of California strawberries—available year round, by the way—might have contributed to putting a ton of carbon dioxide into the atmosphere as it was trucked across the country or even up from Mexico.

   A peripheral argument for buying local: Less packaging. You're not going to find those environmentally costly plastic clam shells or Styrofoam trays at the farmers' market, and more often than not, you won't even find a plastic grocery bag there, since most of us have by now been trained to bring our own shopping bags.

3. Local is almost always cheaper. When the supermarket is charging $4.50 a pound for California tomatoes early in our season, I can usually buy them for half that from local produce sellers who may be trucking them 20 miles or less. As summer progresses, a dozen ears of local GMO-free corn can cost a mere $3, making it hardly worth the effort to grow my own and try to fight off the raccoons, squirrels, corn borers and other pests that are just as eagerly awaiting the exact moment of ripeness.

The obvious question that follows the "buy local" soapbox speech is "What happens when winter comes?"

Good question. If you can't grow oranges where you live, that doesn't mean you shouldn't eat them—they are among the healthiest foods available. So buy them in the winter. We can't grow ginger here, so I buy it freely and happily, knowing it has a host of benefits for our health and knowing it costs the environment to bring it here.

Dried beans, one of our superfoods, take a large amount of space to grow and the yield is paltry. It's much easier (and probably cheaper) to buy them at your local supermarket.

Even if you live in a colder zone, you can grow lettuce in a cold frame during the winter. It usually survives to give you fresh greens in the winter months. Plus, you can always rely on dehydrated and frozen goodies to help you make it through the winter.

There is a delightful story of a family who decided to eat only what could be produced within 100 miles of their home for an entire year. It was a great concept, but in reality, it was extremely difficult because they lived in British Columbia and some things were simply not available, especially in winter. Among the shortfalls: no source of oil for cooking or dressings. Oil is an essential component of our nutrition and, without it, we cannot survive. The wise family of locavores decided an exception had to be made for cooking oil.

We are no longer a society of hunters and gatherers. If we were, we would know enough to put away seeds and nuts and rose hips and dried, pickled, salted and fermented foods to get us through the winter, not only to keep our bellies full, but also to provide the nutrients we so desperately need.

IS ORGANIC BETTER?

This is an issue I've wrestled with for a number of years. Organic foods are invariably more expensive than non-organic. Crop yields are smaller without all the chemicals, but whatever the reason and however great your commitment to support organic farmers, it's hard to stomach paying $5 for a tomato in January.

There is a substantial body of research now that shows that organic foods are more nutritious than conventionally grown foods. That certainly makes sense to me, but sometimes it is simply too much for my budget.

However, there are certain foods for which I make the greatest effort to buy organic. These foods are called The Dirty Dozen, the common foods that carry the heaviest chemical load. Frequently they are foods that we eat unpeeled, which in some cases increases the potential toxin load. For example, since you're not going to eat the thick peel, buying organic oranges is less important than buying organic peaches or strawberries, where so much goodness is in the peel.

Also, if you're a coffee drinker, consider buying organic since coffee beans are among the most pesticide-laden crops in the world, right up there along with cotton. (But that's a subject for another book . . .)

BUY ORGANIC: THE DIRTY DOZEN

Peaches (highest pesticide load)	Cherries
Apples	Kale
Bell peppers	Lettuce
Celery	Grapes
Nectarines	Carrots
Strawberries	Pears

AREN'T SUPPLEMENTS JUST AS GOOD?

It's true, our soils have been depleted of many of their nutrients and commercially produced fruits and vegetables may not be as wealthy in vitamins and minerals as they once were. But if you're growing your own food and know what is going into the soil, there's no reason to believe your veggies aren't giving you optimal nutrition. I know that many people wonder if it wouldn't be easier to pop a few pills and get their nutrients from supplements?

It might be easier, but it probably won't give you the nutrients you might think.

Foods are extremely complex amalgamations of nutrients. Consider the lowly onion. Actually, it deserves a whole lot of respect, as it's one of the most healing foods we know!

Here's what's in the onion you just chopped into your salad:

- Quercetin: anti-histamine and anti-inflammatory

- Allicin: anti-microbial (fights bacterial, viral and fungal infections)

- Sulphoraphane: fights cancer, diabetes and microbial infections

- Chromium: key to the proper metabolism of sugars and fats; essential to optimal brain function

- Vitamin C: boosts immune system function, improves wound healing, strengthens collagen and connective tissue, helps remove cancer-causing nitrosamines from the body and much more.

- Fiber: ushers excess fats from the digestive tract, prevents constipation and hemorrhoids, assists in weight control, and prevents heart disease, cancer, diabetes, diverticular disease, gallstones and kidney stones.

- Manganese: aids in the formation of bones, connective tissue, blood-clotting factors and sex hormones, plays a role in calcium absorption, blood sugar metabolism and fat and carbohydrate metabolism

- Vitamin B6: contributes to the manufacture of the calming brain chemical serotonin, improves immune system function, breaks down carbohydrates, regulates estrogen and progesterone, reduces risk of heart disease

- Tryptophan: natural anti-depressant, lowers blood pressure, reduces hyperactivity in children, relieves restless leg syndrome

- Folate: prevent birth defects, formation of red and white blood cells, maintains and repairs cell, removes homocysteine from blood, lowering risk of heart disease

- Potassium: reduces blood pressure, lowers risk of heart attack and stroke, relieves anxiety, irritability and stress, relieves fatigue

- Copper: promotes proper growth, essential for energy production, red blood cell formation, reduction of cholesterol, important in bone growth, helps regulate heart rhythm, contributes to wound healing connective tissue, eye and hair health

All this and just 60 calories! No fat. Great taste. How does that stack up to a pill? I never heard of an onion pill, but eating an onion is a lot like taking a multi-vitamin.

My point is this: No food is made up of just one nutrient. Not only do we need *all* of these nutrients, scientists are slowly beginning to realize what moms and grandmothers have known since the beginning of time: The whole is greater than the sum of the parts. There is a synergy between these nutrients that makes each one more powerful and enhances all the others.

So get your nutrients from food as much as you can. Don't hesitate to take a multivitamin—you never know if your soil is low on selenium or boron—but look to a healthy diet for most of your nutrients. Conversely, don't think you can eat junk food all day long and make up for it by popping a few strategic supplements. It just doesn't work that way.

FOR THE LOVE OF THE GARDEN

The health benefits of spending time in my garden go far beyond the nutritive value of the foods I grow. Gardening is a wonderful form of exercise. Exercise physiologists say it is at least as effective in burning calories as jogging, but in my humble opinion, it's much more fun!

You'll feel the burn as you lift baskets of compost, till the soil, carry water and pull weeds.

Exposure to fresh air and sunshine also make gardening an effective stress reliever and give my body the chance to manufacture my own free vitamin D. Since I work from home, I can take gardening breaks throughout the day. Spending just ten minutes pulling weeds or pruning an overgrown oregano plant allows my mind to rest and the stress to simply flow into the earth, leaving me refreshed and ready to return to the task at hand with renewed enthusiasm and focus.

Treating your garden as your doctor can make your life full. I know that's true for me.

PART 2

101 Ailments You Can Prevent and Treat with Food

Most of us don't think of the food on plates quite literally as medicine, but when you're finished reading this section, you'll know you can treat and prevent a wide range of ailments simply with powerful healing properties of the fruits of your garden.

ACNE

YOUR GARDEN RX: dried beans, berries, watermelon, walnuts

When you were a teenager, your mom probably told you that chocolate and those yummy greasy French fries caused acne, but for once, she was wrong. Hormone fluctuation is the major cause of acne, which is why it rears its ugly head at puberty often during the menstrual cycle in a woman's childbearing years, and again at menopause if you're a woman, or andropause if you're a man. Stress is also a factor, as can be those harsh products you use in a vain attempt to make the zits go away.

Conventional medicine often treats acne with long courses of antibiotics, a risky plan because it can reduce your body's ability to respond to antibiotics when you really need them—to treat a serious infection, for example.

Your best defense is healthy, clean, hydrated skin plus a few healers from the garden.

Your Garden to the Rescue

Beans are a good source of B vitamins and zinc that nourish your skin and keep it healthy. **Berries**, especially blueberries, raspberries, and cranberries, are rich in phytochemicals that help protect skin cells.

Watermelon rind (that's right) rubbed on your skin may help move the lymph through your skin and keep those zits from erupting. It also exfoliates your skin and adds healthy vitamins A, B, and C, which are absorbed right through your skin.

Walnuts are rich in healthy Omega-3 fatty acids, oils that help keep your skin cells plump and flexible.

ADRENAL FATIGUE

YOUR GARDEN RX: sunflower seeds, parsley, beets and beet greens, wild yam

The adrenals are two tiny glands that sit on top of the kidneys and play a vital role in the manufacture of more than 50 hormones, including the stress hormone cortisol.

When your body loses its ability to respond appropriately to stress, adrenal fatigue sets in. People with adrenal fatigue or a more serious condition called adrenal exhaustion (also called Addison's disease) feel tired, weak, and cold.

Some key signs and symptoms of adrenal fatigue include salt cravings, increased blood sugar under stress, increased PMS, pre-menopausal or menopausal symptoms, low blood pressure, mild depression, lack of energy, decreased ability to handle stress, muscle weakness, absentmindedness, decreased sex drive, mild constipation alternating with diarrhea and many others.

The most effective treatment for adrenal fatigue is stress management.

Conventional medicine treats adrenal fatigue with a variety of hormone and glandular extracts and, in extreme cases, with hydrocortisone, a steroid that can actually make the adrenals weaker rather than stronger.

Your Garden to the Rescue

Sunflower seeds are a great source of the B vitamins that are depleted when we are overstressed.

Parsley is mineral-rich, so it helps restore the natural store of minerals depleted during adrenal fatigue. It is high in vitamin C (300 mg per cup), which promotes the production of stress-reducing hormones.

Beets and beet greens are high in organic sodium, so they can help bring low sodium levels back to normal in order to improve adrenal function.

Broccoli has, among many other nutrients, high levels of pantothenic acid, which promotes the production of calming hormones to neutralize the stress hormones.

RX from Outside Your Garden

Wild yam promotes the natural production of progesterone, another adrenal function that falters with adrenal fatigue.

ALCOHOLISM (*Also see Depression*)

YOUR GARDEN RX: spinach and dark green leafy vegetables, cabbage, asparagus, dried beans, kudzu

Alcoholism is a terrible disease that can cause malnutrition and brain and liver damage as well as emotional turmoil. Primary among the effects of alcoholism is severe thiamine deficiency marked by wasting, appetite loss, nausea and other digestive troubles as well as loss of muscle mass, nerve disorders, and depression.

Since few people recognize they are on their way to alcoholism until they are already in trouble, treatment is more often needed than prevention. During the time of withdrawal from alcohol, it's a good idea to eliminate simple carbohydrates as much as possible, since these sugars are similar to the alcohol sugar and may trigger alcohol cravings.

Most of us know someone who is an alcoholic and we know the toll it can take on families. Treatment is difficult and is of uncertain effectiveness.

Your Garden to the Rescue

Spinach and other **dark green leafy vegetables** and **asparagus** are good sources of folates, a group of B vitamins that are often depleted when someone is alcohol dependent. These foods, eaten freely, can help restore nutritional health.

Cabbage and other brassicas or cruciferous vegetables like broccoli, cauliflower and bok choy help detoxify the system and act as a diuretic to flush out toxins. Cabbage is also an excellent liver tonic, so it may help the liver recover its function.

Dried beans have a high fiber content that will help stabilize blood sugars and reduce alcohol cravings

RX from Outside Your Garden

Kudzu. Unless you're a southerner, you may not be familiar with The Vine That Ate the South, but this Asian native is well known for its ability to reduce alcohol intake. Although you wouldn't grow it in your garden since it is incredibly invasive, kudzu root can be very useful in treating alcoholism. You won't have to dig beside the highway; it's available as a supplement.

ALLERGIES

YOUR GARDEN RX: garlic, onions, apples, chamomile

Allergies are your body's response to what it perceives as an invader. With allergies, your immune system reacts or over-reacts to a stimulus whether it's triggered by a particular food (eggs, corn and peanuts are common food allergens), penicillin, pollen, dust, bee stings, mold, pet dander or latex or some similar substance—even though in reality that stimulus may not be at all threatening to you.

When this happens, your body releases histamine, a chemical that can cause a wide variety of symptoms ranging from hives and frantic itching to sneezing, sinus congestion, swelling, and, in serious cases of food and drug allergies, lowered blood pressure, unconsciousness and even death.

Your Garden to the Rescue

Garlic and **onions** to the rescue, again! Add **apples** in the same category because all three of these common garden foods contain a flavonoid called quercetin, which controls the release of histamines during an allergic reaction. Quercetin also reduces the production of leukotrienes, compounds that cause even more severe inflammation than histamines do.

Chamomile is a daisy-like herb whose flowers make a calming and soothing tea. Chamomile is a source of natural antihistamines and quercetin. It may also be helpful in an anaphylactic (severe allergic reaction) episode, but it should not ever take the place of a visit to the emergency room if you know you are severely allergic to peanuts, bee stings or other allergens and have been exposed to them. Drinking a cup or two of chamomile tea daily can help suppress the histaminic reaction, and over time, may make your allergic reactions less irritating or even help them disappear.

RX from Outside Your Garden

If you're a beekeeper, your own honey may also be helpful. Your allergic reactions may be caused by local pollens, so the honey from bees collecting those pollens may act as the antidote to the perceived immune system threat caused by the allergens. If you don't keep bees, try to find honey made from local pollens not more than a few miles from your home.

ALZHEIMER'S DISEASE, MEMORY LOSS AND DEMENTIA

YOUR GARDEN RX: black-eyed peas, grapes, blueberries, sunflower seeds, spinach, asparagus, celery, garlic, sage

As we age, many of us become a "little forgetful" and for some, the problem is much worse than a little forgetfulness from time to time.

Alzheimer's disease is the most common cause of dementia, and a diagnosis is a terrible blow both to the patient and family. However, there are many foods and herbs that can help.

Your Garden to the Rescue

Black-eyed peas are a good source of B vitamins, especially folic acid, B12 and B6. Eating foods high in those B vitamins is excellent way to reduce high levels of an amino acid called homocysteine that is linked to heart attacks and strokes. Research also shows us that as we age, our B12 levels drop, and memory loss is one of the earliest symptoms of B12 deficiency. So it makes to sense to load up on foods rich in B vitamins, including **lentils, avocados, sunflower seeds, spinach** and **asparagus**.

Red grapes and their powerhouse antioxidant *resveratrol* help keep free radicals from building up the biological equivalent of rust in our systems, including in our brains. In addition to resveratrol, grapes are a good source of a number of nutrients that help thin blood, reduce cell inflammation and protect brain cells.

Blueberries are the king of antioxidants and studies show that blueberries can help improve mental performance, among their many health benefits.

Celery is a rich source of luteolin, a compound that research says may help lower levels of the proteins that create plaque in the brain characteristic of people with Alzheimer's.

Sage has been shown to improve memory, even in young people taking tests as well as in patients with Alzheimer's. Scientists think sage may help acetylcholine production to improve nerve communication that is often lacking in people with various types of dementia.

RX from Outside Your Garden

I can't close this section without mentioning turmeric, the curry spice that I'm sure you won't be growing in your garden, but that has so many health benefits it is considered a superfood. People in India, where turmeric is used in daily cooking, rarely suffer from Alzheimer's. Scientists believe it can prevent the buildup of Alzheimer's-related plaque in the brain.

ANEMIA

YOUR GARDEN RX: potatoes, dried beans, pumpkin, arugula, spinach

Low iron levels in the blood cause the most common type of anemia, but there are other more complicated types. For our purposes here, we'll be talking about iron deficiency anemia that occurs when red blood cells aren't carrying enough life-giving oxygen.

If you've been diagnosed with iron deficiency anemia, most likely you are not getting enough iron in your diet or you are losing blood, perhaps through heavy menstrual periods. You're probably thinking about seafood and red meats as the best sources of iron, but you may be surprised to learn that many foods from your garden are also iron-rich.

In general, adults need about 15 mg of iron a day. It requires special attention to get enough from vegetable sources in an absorbable form, but you can do it. If you're a vegetarian and getting your iron solely from vegetable sources (which include dried beans), you'll find that you'll improve the absorbability of iron by including foods with vitamin C in the same meal.

Your Garden to the Rescue

Potatoes are a good combo vegetable, containing a modest amount of iron (2.8 mg) with vitamin C (20 mg). **Pumpkin** is also a good source of iron, with 1.7 mg per half-cup serving. **Pumpkin seeds** are even better with 4.3 mg per one-ounce serving. **Dried beans** and **lentils** are also good sources of iron.

Spinach and **arugula** and dark green leafy vegetables are also good sources of iron (for those of a certain generation, think of Popeye and his energy-giving can of spinach), minerals and vitamin C.

ANXIETY

YOUR GARDEN RX: lettuce, peaches, raspberries, blueberries, borage, lavender, basil

All of us have experienced anxiety at one time or another. For some of us, it can be debilitating as we scroll through seemingly endless past grievances and possibilities for disaster in the future.

Anxiety can have deep effects on the rest of your system if it keeps your body too long in the fight-or-flight response (see Adrenal Fatigue). It is also frequently the flip side of depression. Severe anxiety is also sometimes called anxiety disorder, post-traumatic stress syndrome (PTSD) or panic disorder. It interferes with sleep and causes high blood pressure and irritability.

Calming foods and herbs will help in the short and long term.

Your Garden to the Rescue

Lettuce has traditionally been used as a calmative, often in juice form. It is considered a natural tranquilizer and also calms stress-related headaches.

Peaches are soothing to the entire nervous system and are helpful for a host of stress-related problems, including digestive issues, skin irritation and heartburn. They may promote healthy sleep.

Nerve-soothing vitamin C and other beneficial nutrients that counteract the excess cortisol released during an anxiety attack are plentiful in **raspberries** and **blueberries**. Teas made from the leaves of these plants are also very soothing.

Foods rich in B-vitamins, including those ever-present **dried beans** and green leafy vegetables like **spinach** and **kale** are excellent to address severe anxiety.

Basil is an age-old calmative that has been used to reduce anxiety, lift spirits and improve concentration. Holy basil, a different variety of the familiar herb usually grown in India, is excellent for soothing anxiety.

APPETITE CONTROL

YOUR GARDEN RX: apples, potatoes, grapes, cabbage, leafy greens like bok choy and arugula

Trying to rein in an over-enthusiastic appetite is extremely difficult. Sometimes stress triggers overeating and sometimes there are lapses in brain chemistry that fail to register when you are full.

Vegetables and fruits high in fiber will really help dial

down your hunger and stay with you long enough for you to feel satisfied for hours.

Your Garden to the Rescue

Not only are **apples** high in fiber, they also contain nutrients that help you feel full quickly and then turn off food cravings for hours.

Potatoes (baked, please, and with a *small* amount of olive oil, butter, sour cream or yogurt, since fats help trigger those fullness hormones) are another great source of fiber, as is **cabbage**.

Grapes have a high sugar content, but just a few will help bring your appetite under control, precisely because of their intense sweetness.

Tangy salad greens like **bok choy, arugula, mesclun** and **endive** stimulate your taste buds, helping you feel satisfied while the fiber actually helps slow the flow of glucose into your bloodstream, keeping blood sugars steady and controlling sugar swings that trigger cravings.

APPETITE LOSS

YOUR GARDEN RX: tomatoes, peaches, apricots, red currants, dill, caraway

Loss of appetite is a symptom of a variety of illnesses, but the most common cause in today's high-pressured society is stress. While some people eat more when they are stressed, others eat less or lose their appetites entirely.

People who are ill or are recovering from an illness often experience loss of appetite, as do frail elderly people.

Lifestyle choices that cause appetite loss include heavy alcohol consumption, smoking and heavy sugar consumption, especially in soft drinks. Low vitamin C levels can cause loss of appetite, so eating foods rich in vitamin C may help.

Small, frequent meals may encourage greater food intake.

Your Garden to the Rescue

Tomatoes and other garden foods high in vitamin C, such as **green peppers**, are often used to stimulate appetite.

Dill has natural calming properties, so adding dill to your foods can help relax you and relieve stress. In addition, its strong flavor can help make food more appetizing.

Caraway, those pungent seeds often found in rye bread, help stimulate appetite by increasing the flow of digestive juices and encourage a better appetite. Chew a few seeds before eating for an appetite stimulant.

Some sources say that tangy fruits like **peaches, apricots** and **red currants** will also stimulate appetite.

ARTHRITIS

Arthritis is divided into osteoarthritis, an inflammatory condition, and rheumatoid arthritis, an autoimmune disease. These two most common types of the disease have very different causes.

OSTEOARTHRITIS

YOUR GARDEN RX: hot peppers, cantaloupe, broccoli, strawberries, bell peppers, grapes

Often called "wear and tear" arthritis, this type of joint pain results from the deterioration of the cartilage, which acts as a cushion in the joints. This can be the result of aging—ironically, it's more prevalent among those who have been very active as runners, tennis players, or athletes of almost any type—and it can also be caused by injury and the gravitational effects of obesity. Osteoarthritis affects as many as 10 percent of Americans. It most commonly occurs in the hips and knees, although it can also be a problem in the neck, spine, elbows, wrists, hands, ankles and feet—virtually any major joint. The deterioration of cushioning between joints leads to stiffness, pain and inflammation. The pain and inflammation cycle can be controlled naturally without the dangerous prescription and over-the-counter drugs, which can have serious side effects. Some foods may actually help re-build damaged cartilage.

Your Garden to the Rescue

Hot peppers can offer fast pain relief because they are loaded with salicylates, anti-inflammatories that act like aspirin, and capsaicin, the actual "heat" of the peppers, which blocks the chemical in nerves that transmits pain. You can get the same effect from eating hot sauces made from peppers and cayenne pepper. Topical poultices made from hot peppers can also be helpful, if you can take the heat!

Vitamin C–rich foods like **cantaloupe, broccoli, strawberries, grapes** and **bell peppers** can also help keep the remaining cartilage strong by reducing inflammation and enhancing production of collagen, which strengthens soft tissue.

Red grapes are an excellent source of resveratrol, quercetin and saponins, all highly effective anti-inflammatories.

RX from Outside Your Garden

Ginger and turmeric are exceptionally powerful anti-inflammatories that you're unlikely to grow in your garden, but will be helpful in relieving the pain caused by inflammation.

RHEUMATOID ARTHRITIS

YOUR GARDEN RX: Green grapes, green beans, celery, cucumbers, lettuce, butternut squash, peas, dried beans

This form of arthritis is an autoimmune disease, which means that the body's defense system attacks its own cartilage as though it is a foreign invader. Rheumatoid arthritis (RA) can be crippling and it is immensely painful. The symptoms of both kinds of arthritis are similar, and the treatments for osteoarthritis sufferers will also be of benefit to those with the immune type. In addition, there is some evidence that rheumatoid arthritis may be aggravated by certain foods. Many people with the disease have been able to determine which foods are their individual "triggers" and eliminate them from their diets. Most commonly, these trigger foods are milk products and gluten.

Your Garden to the Rescue

Green grapes, green beans, celery, cucumbers, lettuce and butternut squash are excellent sources of a pigment called beta-cryptoxanthin, a carotenoid found in brightly colored fruits and vegetables that lowers the risk of rheumatoid arthritis.

In general, it's a good idea to increase your intake of all types anti-inflammatory foods, including berries, pumpkin seeds and flavonoid rich grapes and broccoli if you have been diagnosed with RA.

The zinc found in all kinds of peas and dried beans may also help restore immune system health, helping bring an overactive immune system back into balance.

RX from Outside Your Garden

Going a little afield here, I'm guessing that most of my readers aren't fish farmers or olive grove owners, so you won't literally be growing these foods in your garden, but among the most effective treatments for both major types of arthritis is the regular consumption of inflammation-fighting foods like olive oil and salmon and tuna, part of the traditional Mediterranean diet.

ASTHMA (*Also see Allergies*)

YOUR GARDEN RX: strawberries, broccoli, tomatoes, onions, garlic, horseradish spinach, borage, dill

Acute asthma attacks can be life threatening, so please don't stop the prescription medications your doctor has given you. However, over time you may find your need for inhalers will diminish with the help of foods from your garden. Asthma causes inflammation of the airways (bronchial tubes) making it hard to breathe and causing chronic cough, wheezing and shortness of breath. It can also cause a buildup of mucus in the bronchial tubes, making it harder and harder to breathe. The onset of a full-blown attack when the bronchial tubes spasm is truly frightening and, without emergency care, can be fatal.

Your Garden to the Rescue

Vitamin C is a natural antihistamine, meaning it stops the extreme inflammatory response that triggers the wheezing and runny nose, so eating all foods high in vitamin C will be helpful, including **strawberries, broccoli, tomatoes** and **citrus fruits,** if you're lucky enough to live in a place where you can grow them. Some research also suggests that eating lots of vitamin C-rich foods can reduce the severity of asthma attacks. Note: If you're eating citrus fruits, try squeezing the peels and inhaling the aroma. A substance called limonene, which is found in the citrus peel, helps soothe the airways. You can also eat the peels, but wash them well to be sure to remove any contaminants that might be present.

Onions and **garlic** are rich sources of two major anti-inflammatory and anti-asthmatic compounds, quercetin and cepaene, that can help soothe irritated airways.

If you've ever taken a big breath of **horseradish, wasabi, cayenne** or other spicy foods, you've probably noticed that your airways immediately open up if you've been experiencing any stuffiness. This holds true for asthma as well. I don't recommend regularly inhaling the fumes of these pungent foods, but adding them to salads, or better yet to hot soups and stews, will have the same effect.

Leafy greens like **spinach** are good sources of vitamin E, which helps your body release soothing compounds to relax muscles in the lungs.

Borage is a natural decongestant and expectorant, so it can help reduce the mucus in the airways, and **dill** is a traditional relaxant for the bronchial system.

BACK PAIN (*Also see Arthritis*)

YOUR GARDEN RX: chili peppers, cherries, red grapes, mint.

Back pain is the most common pain complaint among Americans, with about 25% of us saying it regularly affects our work, sleep and ability to function in normal daily activities.

Back pain can have a wide range of causes including injury, muscle spasm, deterioration of joints and nerve entrapment.

Conventional medicine treats back pain either by ignoring it or by prescribing painkillers, muscle relaxants and even antidepressants. Steroid shots are common, and, thankfully, most doctors consider back surgery to be the last resort. All of these treatments carry with them side effects and danger and their effectiveness is variable.

Your Garden to the Rescue

Hot chili peppers are the source of capsaicin, a powerful painkiller that is relatively unique in the plant world because it provides quick relief. In many ways, it works like aspirin without the potentially harmful side effects and it temporarily blocks a compound called "substance P" that transmits pain signals along the nerves to the brain. Hot peppers are best used topically for back pain. You can easily make a salve containing chopped peppers, although eating them and spiking your food with hot sauces made from peppers will also help.

If you make a salve, you'll find that it will burn when you first rub it on your skin. This is perfectly normal, but may be a little unsettling until you adapt to it. Wash your hands carefully afterward to avoid inadvertently rubbing it into your eyes (or somewhere worse).

If your back pain is caused by sports-related muscle injury or spasm, eating tart **cherries** may be preventive because they contain substances that can help protect the *quadratus lumborum*, the muscle most often implicated in lower back pain.

A diet that includes **red grapes** (including moderate consumption of red wine) can be an avenue to pain relief thanks to the anti-inflammatory action of resveratrol, quercetin and saponins.

RX from Outside Your Garden

Ginger and turmeric are anti-inflammatory powerhouses, and so helpful for long-term relief of so many conditions that I recommend keeping them on hand all the time, even though you're probably not growing them in your garden.

Also, I urge you to find a good yoga teacher. Be sure to tell your teacher about your back pain. Yoga, properly done, can be one of the most effective back pain remedies.

BAD BREATH

YOUR GARDEN RX: celery, sage, parsley, fennel

Bad breath isn't a disease, but certainly can be uncomfortable for you and your loved ones. It is often the result of poor oral hygiene and is usually an indicator of gum disease.

Bad breath may also be a symptom of some more serious underlying problem such as kidney failure, liver disease or diabetes. People with chronic respiratory problems often have bad breath because of dry mouth.

We all know that eating certain sulfurous foods like our beloved onions and garlic can also cause temporary bad breath, as can the consumption of alcoholic beverages and dairy foods, especially cheese.

If you improve your oral hygiene and that doesn't relieve your bad breath, see your doctor to find out if there is an underlying cause.

Your Garden to the Rescue

Celery can work like a natural toothbrush since it is so fibrous, so if your bad breath is due to poor oral hygiene, it can help clean that gummy food residue off your teeth. It is an excellent addition to your lunch bag.

Many natural toothpastes contain **sage**, for good reason since it is a good source of menthol, thymol and 1,8-cineole, all known to help sweeten breath.

Chewing on a sprig of **parsley** after a meal can immediately neutralize offensive odors because it is one of the richest sources of chlorophyll, a natural deodorizer. If you're a fan of Indian food like I am, you'll notice that there is often a bowl of **fennel** seeds next to the door to help freshen your breath and to encourage digestion after a meal.

BLADDER INFECTIONS

YOUR GARDEN RX: celery, blueberries, turnips, cranberries, mint, thyme

Bladder infection is largely a women's problem, affecting 20% of us at some time in our lives, most often sexually active women during their childbearing years. If you've ever experienced the burning, constant pressure to urinate, abdominal pain and fever of a bladder infection, you know how unpleasant it can be. Men can experience bladder infections, as well, especially if they have prostate dysfunction.

Conventional medicine usually treats bladder infections, also called urinary cystitis or urinary tract infections, with antibiotics. While you shouldn't let the misery go on for weeks at a time, these natural remedies may give you relief in a matter of days.

Your Garden to the Rescue

Dried herbs that contain cineole or thymol are perhaps the most potent healers of the bladder, because they have bladder-specific antiseptic properties. Fortunately, you can grow most of them in your own garden and they make a delicious tea. Among the best in these categories are all types of **mints, rosemary, fennel, tarragon, basil, thyme** and **oregano**. When you first start to feel that urinary urgency or the faintest burning, a tea containing any or all of these herbs can stop an infection before it takes hold.

Celery is a good source of relief from pain and inflammation as well as a diuretic that relieves fluid buildup.

Cranberries are probably the best-known natural remedy for bladder infection, although most of us probably can't grow them in our gardens. **Blueberries** are a great alternative, with many of the same healing properties of cranberries, including some antibacterial effects.

Turnips are a good source of sulfur compounds that have been historically valued for their urinary health benefits, including helping to relieve fluid buildup and even helping break up kidney stones.

BLOOD SUGAR–HIGH/LOW (*Also see Diabetes*)

YOUR GARDEN RX: beans and legumes, sweet potatoes, cabbage, potatoes, walnuts

Low blood sugar (hypoglycemia) indicates that your body is lacking glucose—its basic fuel source. You can experience hypoglycemia if you haven't eaten for eight hours or more, or if you have a glucose/insulin imbalance or, more likely, if your pancreas's production of glucose-balancing insulin is too high to balance the glucose in your blood. The occasional bout of hypoglycemia usually isn't serious, but repeated episodes can indicate diabetes. Symptoms may be similar to drunkenness, making hypoglycemia especially serious if you are driving.

High blood sugar (hyperglycemia) is an excess of glucose in your bloodstream. While it may seem the opposite of hypoglycemia, the two conditions usually go hand-in-hand and are often precursors of diabetes. Hyperglycemia could be the result of eating too much sugary food, but more likely it indicates that insulin production or absorption is inadequate to balance your sugar intake. Most people with high blood sugar are unaware of it because the symptoms are subtle, but those symptoms can include excessive hunger, thirst, frequent urination and irritability.

It is not unusual for sugar levels to swing between high and low and for sugar cravings to result from low blood sugar.

It's best to eat complex carbohydrates like whole grains and proteins when your sugar is low and to generally center your diet on foods low on the glycemic index, a measure of the effects of carbohydrates on blood sugar levels, to keep your sugars steady and help you avoid a sugar-swing roller coaster. There's a good glycemic index chart at: www.health.harvard.edu/diseases-and-conditions/glycemic _index_and_glycemic_load_for_100_foods.

Because fruit is particularly high in sugar, it is best to avoid high fruit consumption and certainly to avoid juices— which are concentrated fruit sugar and can cause blood sugar swings.

Your Garden to the Rescue

Potatoes, sweet potatoes, all types of dried beans and **legumes, cabbage** and **nuts** are excellent sources of fiber that digest slowly and release their natural sugars into your bloodstream slowly and steadily. They also give you a balancing protein boost.

RX from Outside Your Garden

Several studies show that cinnamon can help balance blood sugar, so adding a teaspoon a day to your morning cereal or stirring it into your tea can be very helpful.

BODY ODOR

YOUR GARDEN RX: spinach, chamomile, parsley

Sweat is the body's natural cooling system. If you didn't sweat, you'd overheat, dehydrate and you could even die of heat stroke. With sweat can come body odor, so for social reasons most of us use commercial deodorants.

Of course, we sweat when we're exposed to warm temperatures or when we exercise, but anxiety and emotional stress can also cause sweating.

Offensive odors are usually caused by bacterial growth in sweat, so frequent bathing with soap and water is all that is needed in most cases. If you are a heavy consumer of onions and garlic, be aware that those foods may actually cause a body odor beyond bad breath, and if you're a heavy drinker, the alcohol can become an offensive part of your sweat.

If possible, avoid commercial antiperspirants that have aluminum chlorhydrate as a principal ingredient. Aluminum has been implicated as an underlying case in many conditions, including Alzheimer's disease and breast cancer.

Your Garden to the Rescue

Chlorophyll helps cleanse you from the inside out, literally binding with toxins and ushering them out of your body. **Parsley, cilantro** and **mints** are all good sources of chlorophyll, so eating them (especially fresh) can give you natural deodorant protection.

Chamomile tea is calming and relaxing, so it can stop nerves that trigger anxiety-related sweating. Some people even use chamomile teabags in the bath or wipe their underarms with them to curb body odor.

Spinach, cucumbers and other foods high in zinc may help restore natural zinc levels if they have become too low, causing, among other things, offensive body odors.

BONE LOSS–LOW BONE MINERAL DENSITY/OSTEOPENIA (*Also see Osteoporosis*)

YOUR GARDEN RX: beans, kale, broccoli, carrots, spinach, potatoes

Bone health is a vital concern for almost everyone as we age, particularly for post-menopausal women. Low bone mass, also called osteopenia, affects 34 million Americans, although many may be unaware of their condition. When low bone mass reaches a critical level, it is called osteoporosis, a serious weakening of the bones that results in bone deterioration and fractures.

With a good diet and exercise program, your goal will be to reverse the loss of bone mass.

As we age, bones lose their minerals and become structurally weaker than when we were young. Abundant research shows that the more active you are as a young person, the greater your bone density and the lower your risk of bone loss as you age. Weight-bearing exercise (walking, jogging, tennis, and so on) is important for everyone, but it is essential to preserve bone strength as you age.

Since bones are composed of a variety of minerals, a diet rich in minerals, not calcium alone, will help keep them strong, as will optimal intakes of vitamins D and K, which enhance absorption of the minerals by the bones.

Your Garden to the Rescue

Calcium-rich foods are part of the equation, but you'll need to balance calcium with other minerals to avoid calcium overload, which won't help your bones at all. **Broccoli** and **kale** are good sources of calcium and they're an excellent source of other essential minerals, like potassium, selenium and the vitamins that help absorb them, including vitamin K.

All **dried beans**—especially dark-colored beans like black beans and dark red kidney beans—are a good source of protein, which helps keep bones strong. In addition, the protein in legumes helps your body form collagen to help hold the minerals in bones.

Vitamin A, like the rich stores found in **carrots** and **spinach**, are important elements of remodeling bones. Too much retinol—an element of vitamin A found in cheese and eggs— can contribute to bone loss, but the healthy carotenoids in **carrots** and **spinach** are the "good guys."

Potatoes are excellent sources of potassium that help alkalize your body, balancing the bone-softening effects of an acidic diet characterized by a diet high in red meat.

RX from Outside Your Garden

Unrefined sea salt contains dozens of trace minerals, many of which are needed for bone strength. To get the best, look for a telltale pinkish color that lets you know all the minerals are intact.

BRONCHITIS

YOUR GARDEN RX: onions and garlic, elderberries, hot peppers, thyme, turnips, kohlrabi, mustard greens

Bronchitis is an inflammation of the main airways to the lungs that often follows a cold or flu. It may be short-lived or it can become a chronic condition. A cough that produces phlegm and produces wheezing, a sore throat, and perhaps even difficulty breathing, chest pain and nasal congestion could be bronchitis.

Children, smokers, people who live with smokers in the house are very susceptible to bronchitis.

Conventional medicine treats bronchitis with antibiotics, but growing evidence shows that although the condition is inflammatory, it is still likely that it's not bacterial, but instead caused by viruses and fungi, against which antibiotics are ineffective.

Your Garden to the Rescue

If you're looking for an antiseptic, a cough suppressant, and a decongestant, you couldn't do much better than **onions** and **garlic**. These potent sulfurous veggies ease coughs and congestion. If you're brave enough, combine two finely chopped onions with two tablespoons of honey. Cover and let it sit overnight and then take a tablespoon to ease congestion.

Elderberries are good antimicrobial foods, meaning you don't need to know if you have a bacterial, fungal or viral infection, because it will help knock them all out.

All sorts of hot peppers—**jalapeños, chilies, habaneros**—help break up congestion, so go for them! They're also a good source of vitamin C, a natural antibiotic. Spicy-hot foods like **mustard greens, horseradish** and **kohlrabi** from the cabbage family, as well as those served piping hot, are very effective at easing congestion.

Thyme is used throughout Europe to stimulate immune function and clear mucus from the lungs and airways.

BRUISES

YOUR GARDEN RX: cabbage leaves, blueberries, arugula, parsley

Bruises are usually the result of an injury that breaks the tiny blood vessels under your skin without breaking the skin. The purple and blue marks are actually pooled blood that will in time be reabsorbed by your body.

Strengthening your blood vessels and the elastic-like collagen in your body will help prevent bruising or make bruising less likely should you have an injury. If you have chronic bruising and fragile skin, you may have a vitamin C deficiency, so C-rich foods will help.

Your Garden to the Rescue

Blueberries, citrus fruits, tomatoes and **sweet peppers** are all rich in vitamin C and will help strengthen the connective tissue to prevent or minimize bruising.

Poultices made from **cabbage** and **arugula** leaves and crushed **parsley** cooked in wine are time-honored remedies for bruises when they're applied as poultices to speed the healing process and disperse the pooled blood beneath the skin. In addition, eating **arugula** and other green leafy vegetables gives you a good amount of vitamin K, a nutrient that may be deficient in people who are prone to easy bruising.

BURNS

YOUR GARDEN RX: chamomile, onions, garlic, cucumber, apples

We don't easily forget the pain of a burn, which can last from minutes to weeks. While there is little we can do to prevent burns except—duh—be a little more careful. Accidents do happen. The immediate first aid for a burn is cool water to stop the burning action through the layers of skin. One thing to avoid: the old home remedy of putting butter on a burn. That actually seals in the heat and can contribute to deeper burning.

Over the long term, while it is healing, you'll want to keep the skin clean and moist.

If the burn is serious, you'll actually see the layers of skin repairing themselves.

Your Garden to the Rescue

In the short term, you'll be looking for nice, cool things to put on your burn. **Cucumbers** immediately come to mind, especially if you've got some in the fridge. They'll not only soothe the sore skin; they'll draw out the heat.

Poultices of **onions** or **garlic** can help cleanse the burn and prevent infection. There is some evidence that onions may even reduce scarring and garlic may help regenerate the damaged skin.

Apples can also help heal burns with a gel-like substance called pectin (it's what makes jelly jell). Just rubbing an apple slice on the burn can help healing, but may not do much for pain.

CANCER PREVENTION

YOUR GARDEN RX: garlic, onions, broccoli, berries (all types), beans, chili peppers, pumpkin seeds, rosemary

There is abundant evidence that a diet rich in all kinds of fruits and vegetables can prevent most types of cancers. That's because as we age, our cells literally start to get a little rusty. Free-radical oxygen molecules attack our cells, much like rust on a car bumper, and mess up the DNA codes that once prompted cells to divide into perfect copies of their parent cells. Among other things, this can cause cancer. Almost all fruits and vegetables are rich sources of antioxidants, so think of them as scrubbing that rust off the bumper.

The National Cancer Institute estimates that one-third of all cancer deaths are related to diet in some way.

There are some powerhouse fruits and vegetables and herbs that not only are study-proven to prevent a wide variety of cancers; some can even slow the growth of existing cancers.

Your Garden to the Rescue

Garlic is often called a superfood because of its multitude of health-giving, even life-saving nutrients. One substance found in garlic, s-allylcysteine, stops cells from becoming cancerous and others, like diallyl-sulfides, actually stop already cancerous cells from dividing, working in ways that are similar to some chemotherapy agents, but are nontoxic. Study after study has shown that people who eat the most garlic have the lowest rates of a variety of cancers, including stomach, colon and liver.

Onions have many of the same sulfur compounds as garlic, with the addition of fructo-oligosaccharides that have a unique ability to knock out bacteria that may cause certain types of gastrointestinal cancers. Onions can slow the growth of breast, colorectal and oral-cavity cancers.

Broccoli and other cruciferous vegetables like cauliflower, cabbage and Brussels sprouts are rich sources of indole-3-carbinols, substances that neutralize the effects of harmful estrogens. That makes them particularly important in preventing breast and other hormonally related cancers.

The sulphoraphane in these vegetables deactivates those dastardly free radicals and helps prevent colon and rectal cancers.

Red grapes are a rich source of resveratrol and ellagic acid, among the most potent antioxidants known. These substances can wipe out the enzymes that encourage cancer cell growth and prevent your immune system from correcting the wild cell growth.

Beans are a low-fat superfood, rich in a variety of nutrients, fiber and protease inhibitors that have been proven to keep normal cells from turning cancerous and prevent cancer cells from growing. Go for the darker-colored dried varieties, like black beans and kidney beans.

Chili peppers like **jalapeños** contain a chemical, capsaicin that can neutralize cancer-causing nitrosamines and may help prevent gastrointestinal cancers.

Berries of all kinds, especially **blueberries**, are good sources of cell-protecting ellagic acid. Ellagic acid not only prevents cellular changes that can lead to cancer, it reduces free-radical damage and helps sweep carcinogens out of your system.

Rosemary can help increase the activity of detoxification enzymes and even slow the development of both breast and skin tumors.

Tomatoes are a source of carotenoids that offer so many health benefits, including lycopene, which has been study-proven to reduce the risk of breast, prostate, pancreatic and colorectal cancers. One study shows that lycopene actually kills mouth cancer cells.

Celery has a unique type of phenolic acids that actually block the action of prostaglandins, hormone-like substances that encourage the growth of cancer cells.

CANKER SORES, COLD SORES

YOUR GARDEN RX: chamomile, sage, raspberries, beets, tomatoes, sprouts

Canker sores or cold sores can have a variety of causes, including the herpes simplex virus, which is usually the culprit in the ones that occur outside your lips.

The ones inside your mouth usually have one of three causes:

1. Irritation from spicy or rough-textured foods

2. Injuries (like biting your lip or tongue, or problems with dental appliances)

3. Stress or chewing the inside of your mouth

If you have a sore caused by the herpes virus, you probably already know that there is no known cure for herpes. However, research shows that foods with significant amounts of the amino acid lysine may diminish the number of herpes outbreaks.

If your sore is due to injury or irritation caused by food or stress, the good news is that it will probably heal on its own in a few days. You can speed healing by swishing a teaspoon of unrefined sea salt in eight ounces of warm water in your mouth two or three times a day.

Your Garden to the Rescue

If it is an external sore: Look for foods rich in lysine and low in arginine to contain the herpes virus. **Beets, tomatoes** and most types of **sprouts** are good suppressors of the herpes virus, so eating them may diminish the number of outbreaks.

You'll want to avoid arginine-rich foods, including chocolate, nuts, caffeine and products made with white flour, because they aggravate the herpes virus.

You'll also do well with immune system-enhancing foods rich in vitamin C, like **strawberries** and **green peppers**.

If the sore is inside your mouth: **Chamomile** tea is a good source of natural painkillers and has a drawing property that can help dry up mouth sores quickly. **Raspberry** root bark or leaf (dried or fresh in a tea) is not only a natural painkiller, it's got three "anti's:" it's antiseptic, anti-inflammatory and antiviral. Sage laves have drawing properties that can help dry up those inflamed mouth sores that you seem to bite over and over again.

RX from Outside Your Garden

For internal or external sores: a milk compress (five seconds on, five seconds off for five minutes, three or four times a day) may help dry up a canker sore or cold sore.

CARPAL TUNNEL SYNDROME
(*Also see Hypothyroidism*)

YOUR GARDEN RX: Pumpkin and sunflower seeds, walnuts

Carpal tunnel syndrome is an inflammatory condition that results from repetitive use of the metacarpals ("fingers" in lay language) and constriction in the nerve tunnel that runs from the fingers through the wrist. It's a disease of our times because it is common among people who use computers and do a great deal of keyboarding. Carpal tunnel syndrome can also be a symptom of hypothyroidism.

Your Garden to the Rescue

Essential fatty acids, like those you find in nuts and seeds like **pumpkin, sunflower** and **walnuts** and in their oils, help counteract inflammatory prostaglandins, minimizing the swelling and relieving the symptoms.

RX from Outside Your Garden

Flaxseed and flaxseed oil are potent sources of essential fatty acids and can help reduce the inflammation of carpal tunnel, although you're unlikely to be growing flaxseed in your garden.

If you use a computer for hours a day, be sure your posture is good (back straight and chin roughly parallel to the floor) and your wrist in neutral position (more or less straight) when you're typing.

CELIAC DISEASE

YOUR GARDEN RX: spinach, potatoes, beans, cantaloupe, tomatoes, sweet potatoes, sunflower seeds

Celiac disease is a hereditary disease that is characterized by extreme sensitivity to gluten in wheat, barley, rye and some other cereal grains, causing severe gastrointestinal upsets.

Happily, modern medicine and natural medicine are on the same page about this one: Avoid products containing gluten, including bread, cakes, pastries, etc. This rigorous dietary constraint has become easier in recent years with a plethora of gluten-free foods on the market due to the increased public awareness of the problem of gluten intolerance as well as higher awareness of the proper treatment of the problem by people who have intolerances, including celiac disease.

Many people who have celiac disease are also lactose intolerant, which means they cannot properly digest dairy products.

Your Garden to the Rescue

If you have celiac disease, you'll be happy to know that virtually anything you grow in your garden (unless you're into growing wheat) is gluten-free and you can eat as much of it as you want. While there is no known cure for celiac disease, it is manageable.

Deficiencies in vitamins A, D, E and K, as well as iron and magnesium, are common among people with celiac disease, so search out foods that have good levels of these essential nutrients for the best results.

Spinach is at the top of that list, as an excellent source of vitamins A, C and K as well as iron. Most leafy greens like **kale, collards** and **Swiss chard** are nearly as good. **Potatoes,** and especially potato flours as an alternative to wheat flours, are usually well tolerated by people with celiac disease.

Cantaloupe and **tomatoes** are great sources of vitamin C and **sweet potatoes** are a great source of vitamin A.

Sunflower seeds are a good source of vitamin E that you can grow in your garden.

Bonus from Your Garden

Did you know that the sun is your best (and cheapest) source of vital vitamin D? Just getting out and weeding your garden for 15 minutes a day—without sunscreen on your arms, shoulders, and legs—will let you absorb enough ultraviolet B (UVB) rays to manufacture all the vitamin D you need without the risk of sunburn even for the fairest skinned people.

CHRONIC FATIGUE SYNDROME AND FIBROMYALGIA

YOUR GARDEN RX: garlic, cabbage, mustard greens, potatoes, rose hips

Chronic fatigue syndrome (CFS) is a terrible hodgepodge of symptoms that leave you feeling utterly drained.

If bed rest does not improve the exhaustion for a period of six months or more, your doctor may be able to arrive at an official diagnosis. Many CFS sufferers spend years going from doctor to doctor before they are diagnosed.

Symptoms can include weakness and muscle pain (also symptoms of fibromyalgia, characterized mainly by extreme sensitivity at certain muscle trigger points), impaired memory, headaches, insomnia and exhaustion following physical exercise, if the exhaustion lasts more than twenty-four hours. In addition to the food recommendations included in this section, look for more advice among the entries for other symptoms you are experiencing.

If you do get a definitive diagnosis, conventional medicine will often treat you with antidepressants and behavioral counseling, since that is about all conventional medicine has to offer.

Your Garden to the Rescue

Your garden has much to offer in terms of relief. **Garlic** has been shown to reduce the symptoms of fatigue from physical exertion and it seems to work for people with CFS as well. Increasing your consumption of foods rich in various forms of B vitamins, like **cabbage, broccoli, cauliflower** and **spinach** will help.

Potatoes and other foods high in potassium and magnesium can help relieve muscle pain and fatigue.

Low levels of a "feel good" brain chemical called dopamine can cause fatigue, so eating **mustard greens** and **watercress**, which are good sources of tyrosine, the amino acid from which dopamine is made by your body, can help relieve the fatigue and low energy.

Research shows that vitamin C is a factor in reducing fatigue, so eating a variety of foods rich in vitamin C can improve your stamina. **Rose hips**, those bud-like remainders of roses after they have bloomed, have very high vitamin C levels. You can dry them and make a make a wonderful tart tea from them. Other C-rich foods are **strawberries, tomatoes, cantaloupe** and **citrus fruits**.

RX from Outside Your Garden

Many people with CFS have low blood pressure. Unrefined sea salt is a good source of the minerals you need, including sodium, to bring your blood pressure and your energy back to normal. Also, you're probably not growing bananas in your garden, but a potassium-rich banana a day can keep the muscle pain away.

COLDS/FLU

YOUR GARDEN RX: elderberries, hot peppers, red peppers, butternut squash, cherries, garlic, onions, mushrooms, sage, echinacea

We all know there is no cure for the common cold and most of us know that colds and flu are caused by viruses, against which antibiotics are useless and may even be dangerous in the long term. Overuse of antibiotics can diminish their effects when you really need them to fight a serious infection, for example.

Doctors tell you to rest, drink lots of fluids and wait for a week or two for the cold or flu to pass. All of that is good advice, but there are foods that will strengthen your immune system so you aren't as likely to get colds or flu, as well as foods and herbs that will help shorten the duration and soften the symptoms if you do get sick.

Your Garden to the Rescue

Let's start with strengthening your immune system to prevent colds and flu. **Onions** and **garlic** are among our best sources of immune system strengthening compounds, including sulfur and allicin. Keep colds and flu away with these powerhouse nutrients.

Foods rich in selenium are also important immune system strengtheners, although most of them are meat and seafood. If you're growing **mushrooms** in your basement, you've got a jump start on beating seasonal colds and flu.

Echinacea has been shown to be helpful in strengthening the immune system, although some studies question its effectiveness.

If you've already got a cold or flu, **hot peppers** and **chili** peppers will help ease the congestion in your head and chest. Some of us masochistically enjoy drinking cayenne pepper tea with lemon and maybe a little bit of honey added when a cold hits.

Elderberries are a powerhouse of natural antiviral compounds, so load up on them if a cold or flu has got you down and out. They reduce inflammation and the muscle aches so common with the flu. In addition, elderberry syrup is an excellent cough remedy. You can buy elderberry syrups, or if you're adventurous here's the simplest recipe I could find:

1. Crush, squeeze and strain about two gallons of very ripe berries. You'll need seven cups of juice.
2. Warm the juice to 165 degrees.
3. Mix juice thoroughly with 14 cups of honey.
4. Put in sterile jars and store in dark place.

Since children under two should not have honey, you can make the syrup by substituting $11^1/_2$ cups of sugar for the honey. You can easily adjust this recipe for a smaller quantity.

If you grow elderberries (a simple task), dry a few in a food dehydrator or low temperature oven against the winter cold season. Like any other dried produce, dried elderberries can be reconstituted by pouring boiling water over them and allowing them to stand for 10–15 minutes.

Sage tea soothes sore throats and calms coughs.

Of course, vitamin C-rich foods are an essential part of your arsenal against colds and flu. **Red** and **green bell peppers, butternut squash** and **cherries** (and all **citrus fruits**, of course) are among the best sources of this vitamin, which has anti-viral properties.

RX from Outside Your Garden

Dark chocolate (oh, yes!) contains theobromine, an excellent cough suppressant. This is enough to make you happy even if you are miserable with a cold.

COLITIS (*Also see Inflammatory Bowel Disease*)

YOUR GARDEN RX: leeks, cabbage, potatoes, squash, pumpkin, zucchini, pears

Colitis, sometimes called ulcerative colitis, affects bowel function and, true, to its name, can cause bleeding ulcers in the colon and rectum. It is often accompanied by severe stomach cramps and violent, bloody diarrhea.

Colitis sufferers usually have periodic flare-ups followed by periods of normal bowel function.

The cause of colitis is unknown, although it often follows an episode of food poisoning or a bacterial infection, oddly enough, in people who have been taking antibiotics to treat an infection.

Colitis can also be caused by a loss of blood supply to the bowel, most frequently due to a contortion of the bowel itself.

Diet is an essential means of treating colitis and most people with the disease have learned that certain foods tend to trigger flare-ups or worsen episodes already in progress. The most common trigger foods are wheat, sugar and dairy products, so eliminating them from your diet is likely to have a positive effect.

Your Garden to the Rescue

You'll want to avoid harsh, acidic or spicy foods for obvious reasons.

Leeks can stop intestinal cramping, gas and bloating. They produce mucilage that coats and soothes the irritated bowel lining.

Cabbage and other cruciferous vegetables like **broccoli** have the same intestinal soothing effect. Cabbage has specifically been used to heal ulcers, as have **squash**, **pumpkin** and **zucchini**.

The mild comforting effect of **potatoes** can help soothe an irritated bowel. Potato juice has traditionally been used as a folk remedy for all types of ulcers.

These foods should be gently poached, perhaps in chicken broth for flavor, without added spices.

Pectin and fiber in pears can help stop diarrhea and the cooling tannins can calm an irritated digestive tract.

CONJUNCTIVITIS (RED EYE/PINK EYE)

YOUR GARDEN RX: blueberry, bilberry, cucumber, chamomile

Conjunctivitis is an inflammation of the conjunctiva, the surface of the eye and the inner surface of the eyelid. It is often caused by a viral infection, but can occasionally be the result of an allergic reaction or a bacterial infection. It is very painful and usually results in an extreme sensitivity to light. There may be a yellow-green mucous discharge from the eye if the inflectional is bacterial.

Modern medicine often treats conjunctivitis with antibiotics, although antibiotics will be ineffective if the cause is viral or allergic. Cold compresses and even cool eyewashes can help ease the inflammation.

Your Garden to the Rescue

Blueberries and **bilberries**, mashed and steeped in water and strained, are a traditional treatment for conjunctivitis. They are rich in vitamins A and C and are a potent source of antioxidants that reduce inflammation and help strengthen the immune response to viral and bacterial invaders.

Cucumbers, especially if they have been in the refrigerator, can be sliced and placed on your eyes for cooling relief. While we're still thinking "cool," a mild wash of **chamomile** tea can help ease the pain.

CONSTIPATION

YOUR GARDEN RX: apples, dried beans, berries, rhubarb, squash

We've all experienced constipation from time to time. The cramping and bloating that accompany the inability to move your bowels can be tiring as well as painful.

Here's one place where conventional medicine and natural medicine agree: Fiber, fiber and more fiber plus lots and lots of water are the best remedies for constipation. Modern medicine diverges by often advising moving things along with stool softeners, laxatives and even enemas.

It's best to avoid laxatives and stool softeners, which can actually impair the return of normal bowel function and, with long-term use, leave you dependent on them to move your bowels. Let nature take her course. Unless you have a serious disease situation, water, fiber and light exercise will usually give you results in a day or two.

Your Garden to the Rescue

Almost all fruits and vegetables are good sources of fiber and water, so enjoy your produce. **Apples** may be your best friends, because they have both soluble and insoluble fiber in the flesh and the skin.

Dried beans are among the best-known sources of fiber and, if you're concerned about the gassiness that accompanies bean eating, add a little ginger when you cook them.

In addition to providing fiber, all kinds of **berries** prevent bile acid from converting to cancer-causing compounds, thus promoting good health on several fronts.

Elderberries are among the most potent natural laxatives, but **blackberries, blueberries** and **strawberries** are also good.

Rhubarb is an excellent source of insoluble fiber with a natural laxative effect. Dark green **winter squashes** also have many of the same effects.

RX from Outside Your Garden

Dehydration is a frequent cause of constipation, so drink lots and lots of water. To determine how much water you need, experts recommend dividing your body weight by two and multiplying by an ounce a day. In other words, if you weigh 150 pounds, you need at least 75 ounces of water every day. Most doctors say you can't include the moisture in fruits and vegetables in your water intake. Fluids like soft drinks and caffeinated beverages are actually dehydrating, so they don't count either.

COPD (Chronic Obstructive Pulmonary Disease; Includes Emphysema and Chronic Obstructive Bronchitis)

YOUR GARDEN RX: winter squash, green peppers, strawberries, carrots, sweet potatoes, walnuts, sunflower seeds

COPD encompasses emphysema, chronic bronchitis and chronic asthmatic bronchitis, diseases characterized by damage to the airways and air sacs in the lungs that cause breathing to become difficult. COPD is most often caused by cigarette smoking. Symptoms usually worsen over time. Conventional medicine treats COPD with steroids.

Your Garden to the Rescue

There is a wide range of delicious **winter squashes**, like Hubbard and butternut, and all of them are rich in lung-healthy vitamin C and beta-carotene. Toxicologists at the

EPA confirm that people with the highest levels of vitamin C in their blood have the lowest risk of lung diseases. That's because vitamin C is a strong antioxidant that helps neutralize lung damage caused by environmental toxins like air pollution and cigarette smoke. It may also slow the progression of COPD.

Other foods high in C like **green peppers, strawberries** and, of course, citrus fruits will help protect you.

Carrots and **sweet potatoes** are other good sources of beta-carotene.

Pump up your consumption of nuts, like **walnuts**, and seeds, like **sunflower seeds**, for the vitamin E that helps prevent oxidative damage as well.

COUGH

YOUR GARDEN RX: elderberries, chili peppers, horseradish, peppermint

We've all experienced wracking coughs that seem to linger on long past the end of a common cold and keep us from sleeping. That's probably why we spend billions of dollars a year trying to quiet those pesky coughs.

While coughs are usually part of the annoyance of a cold, they can also be a sign of bronchitis or sinusitis.

Your Garden to the Rescue

Gargle some strong peppermint tea and take advantage of its natural cough suppressants and irritant soothers.

Elderberries are among my favorite remedies for colds and whenever my immune system needs a boost, but they are equally effective against coughs when you make them into a berry-sweetened syrup, which is also effective against allergies and sinus inflammation. (See colds and flu for elderberry syrup recipe)

If you're brave, try eating some **chili peppers** to help thin the mucus and reduce chest congestion. If you're even braver, try some **horseradish** for its phlegm-thinning properties.

RX from Outside Your Garden

Try any of these options to find relief from a cough:

- Suck on a clove
- Take a spoonful of honey
- Brew a cup of ginger tea
- Sip a bowl of homemade chicken soup
- Best of all, eat a piece of good dark chocolate

CROHN'S DISEASE (Also see Colitis)

YOUR GARDEN RX: potatoes, sweet potatoes, squash, applesauce

Similar to ulcerative colitis, Crohn's disease most often affects the lower end of the small intestine and results in many of the same symptoms as colitis: diarrhea and abdominal cramping. Crohn's sometimes causes intestinal blockages, which can be life threatening.

People with Crohn's are usually advised to avoid high-fiber and fatty foods. Because there may be a food sensitivity component to Crohn's, it's a good idea to isolate certain foods and see if they cause a flare-up. The most common triggers are wheat and dairy products.

People with Crohn's may have vitamin and mineral deficiencies because of chronic diarrhea.

Your Garden to the Rescue

Most people with Crohn's are advised to avoid raw fruits and vegetables. Gentle foods like baked **potatoes** (avoid the fiber-rich skins during a flare-up), **sweet potatoes** and steamed **squash** are nutrient-packed and gentle on the digestive tract, as are **carrots, beets** and **green** and **yellow beans**.

Applesauce will also give you the pectin that soothes the mucosa of the intestinal tract.

CUTS, SORES

YOUR GARDEN RX: garlic, thyme, plantain, spinach

Stopping the bleeding should always be the first concern when you get a cut. The second is to prevent infection; and the third is to promote healing.

For the most part, you don't need to succumb to the doctor's wish to give you antibiotics and/or a tetanus shot. That's not necessary in most cases, unless there is contact with rusty metal or legitimate reason to fear serious bacterial contamination.

Generally, keep the cut clean and covered and it will heal in a few days.

Fortunately, your garden offers many ways to clean and heal that cut.

Your Garden to the Rescue

Here we go with **garlic** again: It's one of nature's most powerful antiseptics, so putting a garlic poultice on the cut will help draw out dirt and bacteria. **Thyme** and **plantain** (that wide-leafed weedy thing that is probably growing in your driveway or somewhere in your yard) are also powerful antibacterials.

For the healing process itself, you can't beat several big spinach salads for the increased zinc you'll get to help remodel your skin.

RX from Outside Your Garden

Honey is a great antibacterial that can act as a natural bandage, since it will seal the cut as it dries.

CYSTS (Cervical and Ovarian)

YOUR GARDEN RX: onions, garlic, blueberries, milk thistle, dandelion leaves, burdock and yellow dock

Cervical and ovarian cysts are most often harmless growths. Ovarian cysts can grow inside or outside the ovaries. Cervical cysts are just as they might seem—small pockets, usually of mucus, that grow inside the cervix.

Your Garden to the Rescue

Foods that help detoxify the body can be helpful in reducing the incidence of ovarian and cervical cysts. **Onions, garlic** and **blueberries** are among the most potent detoxifying foods and the antimicrobial properties of onions and garlic may also help stop any secondary infection. Detoxifying herbs, such as **milk thistle**, can also be helpful. You're not likely to be actively cultivating so-called "weeds" like dandelions, burdock and yellow dock, but you'll undoubtedly find these helpful detoxifiers nearby.

DEHYDRATION

YOUR GARDEN RX: watermelon, cantaloupe, pears, peaches, tomatoes

If you're dehydrated, you need water, plain and simple.

Dehydration can cause a wide variety of health problems, including muscle cramping, weakness, headache and in serious cases, convulsions, heart failure, kidney failure and death.

In severe cases, you must be hospitalized and your fluid balance restored intravenously.

If you are dehydrated, you need to increase your water consumption until the symptoms disappear and then adopt a regimen of drinking water daily. If plain water is distasteful to you, add a little squeeze of lemon, a sprig of peppermint, a slice of cucumber or a bit of ginger.

Your Garden to the Rescue

While water is always the best remedy, lots of watery vegetables and fruits and juices will help you get back the deficit and even help replace some of your lost electrolytes.

Think about watery foods like **watermelon, cantaloupe, pears, peaches** and **tomatoes**. When you add in the A and C vitamins and rich mineral content, these foods will help rehydrate you and keep you hydrated.

DEPRESSION

YOUR GARDEN RX: kale, spinach, dried beans, mushrooms, sunflower seeds, oregano, garlic and onions

There are several types of depression. These are the most common:

- Mild moodiness from time to time

- Winter blues (often related to vitamin D shortfalls in winter)

- Holiday- or anniversary-related sadness, especially in remembrance of times past and loved ones who are no longer here

- Full-blown moderate or even major depression

While there are definitely psychological components of depression, most clinical depression is caused by shortfalls in certain brain chemicals called neurotransmitters. You've probably heard of serotonin, dopamine and norepinephrine, the Big Three "feel-better" neurotransmitters. Low levels of any of these can cause depression, cravings, addiction, obesity, insomnia and other unpleasant health side effects.

Modern medicine likes to prescribe antidepressants for just about anyone who complains of sadness, despite the fact that they don't work at all for half the people who take them. There is often a price for those who do get positive results, in the form of serious side effects.

Fortunately, your garden has several good answers and natural medicine has even more.

Your Garden to the Rescue

A number of nutrients, including B and C vitamins and selenium, give your body the building blocks to manufacture the neurotransmitters that will lift your mood.

Green leafy vegetables like **kale, spinach** and dark green **lettuces** (not iceberg; that has almost no nutritional value), sunflower seeds and **dried beans** are excellent sources of vitamin B6, also known as folate, the building block for serotonin. This is especially important if you are taking folate-depleting birth control pills or hormone replacement.

Brazil nuts are by far the best source of selenium, a mineral that plays a key role in depression. **Mushrooms**, which you can grow in your basement, are among the few vegetable sources of selenium. **Oregano** has much the same effect.

Although **onions** and **garlic** are commonly associated with relief from depression, they contain substances that act just like the old-time antidepressant medications called MAO-inhibitors, which often are more effective than the newer medicines

RX from Outside Your Garden

Chocolate has more than 300 brain-altering compounds that can raise your spirits. No wonder we love it so much! If you haven't gotten the message by now, I love chocolate and I am very glad that it is good for us! Be sure to go for good quality dark chocolate. Milk chocolate is loaded with sugar.

DIABETES (*Also see Obesity/Weight Control, Blood Sugar, Heart Problems*)

YOUR GARDEN RX: dried beans, green beans, onions and garlic, sweet potatoes, blueberries, sunflower and pumpkin seeds

Diabetes is one of the most widespread and insidious diseases known to the modern world. Type 2 diabetes, the most common form, generally begins in adulthood, although it is becoming disturbingly common in teenagers and even pre-teens. That's because 95% of people with Type 2 diabetes are obese.

With today's epidemic of obesity, it's not surprising that

more and more people will be affected by this disease, which comes from the body's inability to use the insulin it produces to balance blood sugar from our diets.

It also opens you to a high risk of other serious diseases, including heart disease, kidney failure, macular degeneration (an eye condition that can cause blindness) and circulatory problems that can lead to amputations.

Conventional medicine chooses to treat most people with Type 2 diabetes as though they have already had a heart attack, largely because their risk of a heart attack is very high, about triple that of non-diabetics.

Diabetes demands strict attention to diet and restricting the intake of simple sugars, including excessive amounts of fruit. It pretty much bans fruit juice altogether. Fruit in moderate amounts (1–2 pieces per day) is definitely allowed on a diabetic diet, but juices are the sources of far too much concentrated fruit sugar. For example, you might eat an orange or even two. But you wouldn't eat six or eight oranges— that's how many are in a typical glass of orange juice. Read the label and you'll see how much sugar is in juice.

Today's dietary guidelines for people with diabetes no longer prohibit sugary foods, instead emphasizing a healthy diet and exercise program that is much more realistic than complete avoidance of simple sugars.

Exercise is very important because the energy used by muscles enhances the body's ability to use insulin and improves blood sugar balance.

Conventional medicine treats diabetes with a wide range of pharmaceuticals. People with diabetes often take multiple medications and sometimes insulin to control blood sugar as well as drugs to control cholesterol levels and blood pressure, and to support the hearts, kidneys, and eyes.

There is no cure for diabetes. However, choosing the

healthiest possible lifestyle can lower your need for medications, and perhaps even eliminate the need for some as you begin to control your blood sugar more effectively.

Weight control is at the heart of almost all diabetes treatment plans, since so many people with diabetes are obese.

Your Garden to the Rescue

Because weight control is probably your goal, almost everything in your garden is good for you. Remember, you'll need to limit the intake of fruit (most docs say no more than two servings a day) and some starchy veggies like potatoes.

But you can load up on low-sugar high-energy foods like dark green leafy veggies (**kale, collards, dark green lettuces, spinach**).

Foods high in fiber, like our favorite **dried beans**, slow down the digestive process and ration the entry of sugars into your system. The high fiber content in **sweet potatoes** and their unique levels of chlorogenic acid also help control blood sugars.

Onions are great for diabetics because they contain chromium, antioxidants and flavonoids that can result in major blood sugar reduction when you eat two or more ounces per day. They can also help raise your metabolic rate when eaten raw, addressing the obesity problem.

Garlic, another perennial favorite, helps lower blood sugar and encourages the pancreas to produce more insulin.

All kinds of nuts and avocados contain good fats that help lower insulin resistance.

RX from Outside Your Garden

Many studies show that cinnamon helps lower blood sugar.

Choose complex carbohydrates that absorb their sugars slowly into your bloodstream, such as brown rice and baked goods made with whole grains (not just whole wheat).

DIARRHEA

YOUR GARDEN RX: apples, potatoes, carrots, garlic, onions, leeks

Almost everyone is affected by diarrhea from time to time. Although it's most commonly caused by a virus or food sensitivity, it can also be caused by a bacteria attached to food (food poisoning).

Most cases of diarrhea disappear in a day or two without treatment because we have large colonies of helpful bacteria in our digestive tracts that can fight off pathogens without too much trouble.

However, diarrhea caused by other illnesses (colitis or inflammatory bowel disease, for example) or episodes that last more than a few days can be serious, primarily because you're losing large amounts of fluid from your system and you're at risk of dehydration. Children are especially vulnerable to dehydration from diarrhea and can be at risk of serious illness in as little as one day.

Your Garden to the Rescue

Avoid most raw fruits and vegetables for a few days and go with lightly steamed gentle veggies (asparagus, peeled zucchini, green beans, peas), or a baked **potato** and maybe a little homemade **applesauce** for the pectin that helps control diarrhea.

Carrots can help soothe an irritated digestive tract and help replace vital nutrients lost due to diarrhea.

Garlic, onions and leeks are natural sources of probiotics that naturally balance your out-of-whack intestinal micro-organisms.

RX from Outside Your Garden

Try the **BRAT** diet: Banana, (brown) Rice, Applesauce and (whole grain) Toast

DIVERTICULITIS (*Also see Constipation*)

YOUR GARDEN RX: apples, dried beans, chamomile, peppermint, thyme

Sometimes small particles of food become trapped in the naturally occurring diverticula or little pouch-like projections in the large intestine. When this happens, the diverticula become inflamed and can cause a painful episode called diverticulitis. Constipation often goes hand-in-hand with diverticulitis.

Seeds, nuts and small particles of food like corn, tomato seeds and celery strings are most likely to be trapped in the diverticula, so it's a good idea to avoid them if you have experienced this problem.

In general, people with diverticulitis need a high-fiber diet and for that, it's only a short trip to your garden.

Your Garden to the Rescue

Apples may be your number one tool against diverticulitis because they are sources of pectin and soluble and insoluble fiber, an excellent pairing to soothe the irritated digestive tract and to usher food through your intestines without causing problems.

Other high-fiber foods, like **dried beans** (cooked with a carrot and perhaps an onion to help keep down the gas and bloating) will also help in the long run after an acute attack has passed.

Herbs that soothe our digestive tract can also offer relief, including **peppermint, chamomile** and **thyme**. Peppermint has loads of anti-inflammatory compounds, painkillers and sedatives. It should be part of your garden and part of everyone's medicinal arsenal.

DRY SKIN

YOUR GARDEN RX: sunflower and pumpkin seeds, carrots, sweet potatoes, green peppers, strawberries

Dry skin is most often caused by overexposure to sun, dry indoor air or a diet too low in fat. We all need the good fats that come from seed and nut oils. Dry skin can be one of the first signs that we're short on good fats. That shortage can have far-reaching consequences, including heart disease and stroke.

Thyroid disease and other endocrine disorders can also cause dry skin, so if there isn't a logical explanation for your dry skin, you might want to have your thyroid function checked.

Your Garden to the Rescue

Pumpkin and **sunflower seeds** contain healthy oils, and they're a good source of skin-healthy vitamin E. If you're lucky enough to be able to grow nuts, you'll find their natural oils help to moisturize your skin as well.

Vitamin C is an internal skin moisturizer often recommended by dermatologists, so C-rich foods like green **peppers, strawberries** and citrus fruits will certainly help.

Carrots and sweet potatoes are also good sources of beta-carotene, a form of vitamin A with strong antioxidant properties that helps protect your skin from sun damage.

RX from Outside Your Garden

Avocados are an excellent form of skin-healthy fat, as are fish like salmon, mackerel, and tuna.

EAR INFECTIONS

YOUR GARDEN RX: garlic, onions, oregano

Ear infections can have a wide range of causes, although the vast majority are caused by a cold virus that migrates into the Eustachian tubes in the ears. Ear infections are most common in children, but adults can also get earaches and ear infections from viruses as well as from earwax compaction, accumulation of water in the ear (known as swimmer's ear), and unequal pressure due to altitude changes (common among scuba divers). In children, food allergies, particularly to dairy products, can be a factor in recurring ear infections, so it might be worthwhile to eliminate dairy products from the diet to see if the condition improves.

Your Garden to the Rescue

Garlic, and onions to a somewhat lesser degree, have powerful antimicrobial sulfur compounds that can knock out viruses as well as bacterial and fungal infections, which means you don't have to know what caused the infections to get relief. You can eat your onions and garlic for a systemic inoculation of those antimicrobial benefits or you can squeeze 2–3 cloves of garlic into two tablespoons of olive oil (use a garlic press), let it infuse for a day, strain, warm it slightly and drop a few droppersful into your ear. **Oregano**, which also has excellent antimicrobial properties, can be infused in oil in a similar way. Loosely pack a jar with wash and dried herb, let it sit for six weeks and then strain and store in a dark place. Strain the oil, warm a small amount, and introduce a few drops into the ear. You should lie on your side when infusing oil into an ear, remain in position for 5–10 minutes, then turn over and drain the oil out of the ear onto a paper towel or tissue. DO not dig with a cotton bud.

RX from Outside Your Garden

Hydrogen peroxide was Grandma's remedy for earaches, and it continues to serve my family and me well today. Lie on your side with a towel under your head to catch any drips and, using an eyedropper, drip six to eight drops of peroxide into your ear and then wait for two or three minutes. The fizzing sound tells you it's working. Then turn over and let it drain out onto a paper towel or tissue. Just for good measure, be sure to treat the other ear, even if you don't have any symptoms.

ECZEMA (*Also see Allergies, Dry Skin*)

YOUR GARDEN RX: potatoes, chili peppers, dried beans

Eczema is a painful itchy, scaly rash, often one of long duration, most often caused by a food or chemical sensitivity, and sometimes by an overactive immune response like those that cause allergies.

While some of the usual suspects like wheat and dairy allergies can be triggers, eczema may also be a response to eggs, seafood, citrus fruits, bath soaps, laundry detergents, nickel in earrings or other jewelry, wool, animal dander, cold weather and even stress.

While there can be a variety of symptoms severe itching is almost always part of eczema, and sufferers often scratch their skin raw. When this happens, secondary infection is a risk.

Conventional medicine usually treats people with eczema with long-term hydrocortisone creams. This is a steroid that can cause serious health problems, so if you can manage your eczema without it, you'll be much better off.

The FDA has also approved two prescription creams, both of which carry the highest level of warnings about health risks.

Your Garden to the Rescue

Foods high in vitamin B6, also called folates, including **potatoes, chili peppers** and **dried beans** can offer relief to eczema sufferers. Keeping your skin moist eases the itching, so the recommendations for dry skin may also help, including sunflower and pumpkin seeds for vitamin E and citrus fruits for vitamin C if you're not sensitive to them.

EYESIGHT DETERIORATION

YOUR GARDEN RX: sweet potatoes, carrots, kale, spinach, melons, tomatoes, potatoes, dried beans

Your eyesight might deteriorate for a number of reasons: glaucoma, cataracts, macular degeneration—all of them eye diseases related to aging.

Conventional medicine treats cataracts with surgery and other eye diseases with a variety of pharmaceuticals.

The foods you consume can go a long way toward preventing eye problems and keeping your eyesight healthy.

Your Garden to the Rescue

Vitamin A is essential for eye health, particularly to improve night vision and to preserve eyesight. Your body converts the beta carotene in foods to vitamin A, so look for a lot of bright orange-colored foods like **carrots, sweet potatoes** and **cantaloupe** and dark green leafy veggies like **kale** and **spinach** to improve your eyesight. Since most macular degeneration is caused by Type 2 diabetes, low glycemic index **sweet potatoes** are an ideal food for diabetics.

Lycopene, a particular type of carotenoid found in ripe red **tomatoes,** has been proven to prevent cataracts and macular degeneration.

Potatoes and other foods rich in B vitamins will help preserve your eyesight, as will vitamin E–rich **green leafy vegetables** and **sunflower** and **pumpkin seeds.**

FEVER

YOUR GARDEN RX: blackberries, raspberries, blueberries, feverfew, borage, calendula

A fever is nature's way of fighting an infection by raising the body temperature and creating an inhospitable environment for disease-causing microorganisms.

Normal human body temperature is 98.6°F and, while any elevation from that baseline could be considered a fever, treatment isn't required until the temperature exceeds 100.4°F.

It's easy to see why a mild fever is a good thing and probably shouldn't be treated, since the fever indicates that the immune system is doing its job of fighting disease.

However, a fever that gets too high can be dangerous and cause convulsions and delirium. Conventional medicine usually uses aspirin to treat a mild fever and encourages increasing fluid intake. Antibiotics may be used to treat the underlying infection if there is a dangerous fever.

Your Garden to the Rescue

The common garden **berries**—blackberries, blueberries and raspberries—are all good sources of vitamin C, which has some natural antibiotic properties. They are also astringent, so they draw out the viral causes of colds, flu, sinusitis and chest infection that are usually the triggers for a fever. Berries are also a good source of salicylic acid, the pain-relieving and fever-reducing ingredient in aspirin. **Blueberries** are a good source of anthocyanins, which help your body fight infections.

Feverfew has traditionally been used to relieve headaches, but as its name suggests, feverfew is an excellent fever reducer.

Borage is a diuretic and helps increase sweat production, helping cleanse the toxins and doing the work of the fever without the dangers. **Calendula**, with its daisy-like flowers, is an astringent and an antiseptic with a rich dose of carotenoids thrown in to help fight infections of all types, even fungal infections.

FLATULENCE

YOUR GARDEN RX: leeks, dill, fennel, peppermint

Gas is a natural product of digestion and *all* of us produce it, no matter how much we may deny it. Gas is actually a sign your digestive system is working correctly.

However, gas can be socially unacceptable. If you eat lots of healthy gas-producing foods like dried beans, cabbage and cucumbers, don't give up the good foods; just neutral-ize the gas.

Your Garden to the Rescue

It may seem counter-intuitive, but "stinky" foods in the onion family, particularly leeks, help re-establish the normal intes-tinal microorganisms to relieve the bloating and cramping that can come from foods that are fermenting in the gut. **Leeks** can also stimulate digestion and ease constipation.

Dill, fennel and **peppermint** belong to a class of herbs called carminatives, which literally means "anti-gas." All of them ease digestive upsets.

RX from Outside Your Garden

Dandelion roots have wonderful anti-gas properties—most of us can find them right in our own backyards—and yogurt contains the live bacteria to help restore the normal microor-ganisms that live in your digestive tract.

FOOD POISONING

YOUR GARDEN RX: garlic and onions, mint, raspberry- and blackberry-leaf tea

Food poisoning results from the consumption of contami-nated food or water. Despite the media attention to food poisoning that occasionally occurs in restaurants, most cases of food poisoning are caused by improper food handling at home. It's usually characterized by abdominal cramping, vom-iting and diarrhea. Warning: If severe symptoms continue for more than two days or if a group of people who ate or drank the same things become ill, or if the symptoms take place in a child under the age of two, seek medical attention.

Your Garden to the Rescue

The first remedy is water, which isn't precisely from your garden, but is essential to preventing the dehydration that can take place after the vomiting and diarrhea that accompany food poisoning. The antimicrobial powers of **garlic** and **onions** may be able to neutralize the bacteria causing the problem. Mint teas will help soothe your stomach and stop the spasms, while **blackberry** and **raspberry** leaf teas are not only helpful in reducing the nausea and diarrhea, but can also help re-establish the mucosal coating in the stomach.

Gallstones (*Also see Heart Problems: Cholesterol*)

YOUR GARDEN RX: radishes, beet greens, dandelion

While gallstones—small lumps in the gallbladder—are not directly related to high cholesterol, they do result from a diet too rich in fat and cholesterol. This "gravel" can cause extreme pain in your right side in the upper or middle abdomen. Conventional medicine usually treats gallstones with drugs that dissolve the stones or with surgery.

Your Garden to the Rescue

Radishes are the source of a variety of fat-reducing digestive enzymes that help the gallbladder increase its bile production and soothe irritated bile ducts, preventing the formation of gallstones. **Beet greens** are good sources of betaine, a bile stimulator and simultaneous diluter of bile that helps bile move more easily though the ducts. **Dandelion** leaf tea or greens eaten raw in salads have also been shown to increase bile flow and improve the body's ability to process fat and cholesterol.

GUM DISEASE (Gingivitis or Periodontal Disease)

YOUR GARDEN RX: strawberries, broccoli, bell peppers, tomatoes

Gum inflammation and infection are almost always a result of poor diet. Gum disease is one of the symptoms of scurvy or vitamin C deficiency, which is much more common today than most medical practitioners care to admit, especially among elderly people whose vitamin C consumption and absorption are less than adequate. Gum disease often is the result.

The Standard American Diet (SAD) of processed foods, sugar and nutritionally void "foods" is largely responsible for our vitamin deficiencies and the diseases that result from them.

While conventional medicine prefers to treat gum disease with complicated, painful, and expensive dental work and antibiotics, eating enough of the healthy produce from your garden can prevent gum disease and even treat it if you have a mild case.

Your Garden to the Rescue

Almost everything in your garden will help promote healthier gums, but foods that are high in vitamin C, including **strawberries, broccoli, bell peppers** and **tomatoes**, will be exceptionally helpful. Drinking a little **rose hip** tea and swishing it around in your mouth before you swallow can also help.

Not only do all of these boost levels of this all-important nutrient in your body, they boost immune system function and act as a natural antibiotic to help fight the infection and inflammation in your gums.

HAIR PROBLEMS

YOUR GARDEN RX: cucumbers, spinach, watermelon, green peppers, dried beans

Hair problems can manifest in a wide variety of ways from brittle, dry hair to thinning and baldness, dandruff and other scalp issues. While dandruff and scalp rashes are most likely indicative of a skin problem, hair itself is made of keratin, a type of protein.

The main nutrient sources for hair include calcium, magnesium, manganese, silicon, iron, and selenium, as well as vitamins A, B6, and C. If you have hair problems, they may signal a basic nutrient deficiency.

Dry, brittle hair is also a symptom of thyroid disorders and hormone imbalances, so if basic dietary changes don't improve the situation, ask your doctor about diagnostic tests.

Your Garden to the Rescue

Cucumbers offer excellent nutrition for your hair, whether you eat them for their abundant mineral content or grate them and wear them on your head for a few minutes to nourish your skin, improve circulation to your scalp, and ease itchiness. However, if you're wearing them on your head, I suggest you don't answer the door or Facetime calls!

Other foods high in minerals and specifically rich in vitamins to help your hair include **bell peppers** for vitamin C, **spinach** for vitamin A, **watermelon** for vitamin B6 and **dried beans** for biotin and zinc.

HEADACHE, MIGRAINE (*Also see Headache, Stress*)

YOUR GARDEN RX: garlic, spinach, sunflower seeds, feverfew, mint, valerian

Migraines are debilitating forms of headache that affect about 10% of us and are more common in women than in men. It has long been suggested there is a hormonal component to migraines, although the headache pattern is highly individual.

Known migraine triggers include:

- Red wine

- Chocolate

- Cheese

- Foods that contain nitrites (such as hot dogs and deli meats)

- Food that contains MSG (monosodium glutamate), especially Chinese food

- Flashing lights

- Weather changes

- Certain odors, particularly perfumes

- Hormone swings

- Stress

By keeping a journal, you'll be able to get a good handle on your triggers and avoid them.

Yes, stress can cause migraines as well as tension headaches. The primary difference between a migraine and a tension headache is that in addition to the crushing head pain, migraines usually are accompanied by nausea and vomiting and are often signaled by an "aura" or a warning signal that may include disturbances in vision or specific smells.

Most migraines are believed to have a vascular element, meaning that blood vessels are either contracting or spasming, contributing to the pain.

Your Garden to the Rescue

Magnesium and vitamin B6 have been shown to stop migraines and perhaps even to prevent them, so eating magnesium- and B6-rich foods like **spinach** and **pumpkin seeds** may help.

Garlic helps thin blood and can stop migraines due to narrowed blood vessels.

Feverfew, mint and **valerian** can all help when a migraine strikes. Feverfew, traditionally used in Europe for headache relief, has painkilling and anti-inflammatory effects that can help migraine sufferers when other methods fail. Mint will help calm a queasy stomach, and valerian will help you sleep and relieve tension.

RX from Outside Your Garden

Ginger can really relieve the inflammation, the spasms, and the blood vessel constriction and dilation that sparks migraines.

HEADACHE, STRESS (*Also see Headache, Migraine*)

YOUR GARDEN RX: blueberries, tomatoes, bell peppers, chamomile, catnip

The vast majority (about 90 percent) of all headaches are related to stress and are triggered by tightening of the muscles of your neck and scalp.

Stress headaches can have a number of causes, including the obvious: emotional or mental stress, depression and fatigue. There can also be less obvious causes: hunger, over-exertion and poor posture.

Chronic tension headaches can occur at regular intervals, sometimes even on a daily basis, and can last anywhere from a few minutes to days on end.

Conventional medicine treats headaches either by ignoring them and suggesting they are "all in your head" (they are—quite literally) or by going overboard with prescription painkillers that can be addicting and have a host of harmful side effects. There are even headaches that are caused by taking too many medications to treat headaches.

Your Garden to the Rescue

Blueberries are a natural source of pain-relieving salicylic acid, a close cousin to the pain-relieving ingredient in aspirin. **Green peppers, tomatoes** and **cantaloupes** are also good sources of salicylic acid.

Better yet, try preventing a headache with a cup of calming **chamomile** or **catnip** tea. (I promise the catnip tea won't make you goofy like it does your cat.)

HEARTBURN

YOUR GARDEN RX: apples, peaches, lettuces and spinach, carrots, fennel seeds, lemon grass, chamomile.

More formally known as GERD (Gastro esophageal reflux disease) is widely believed, even by many doctors, to be caused by excess acid production in the stomach that then splashes up into the esophagus, causing intense pain. In fact, it is not caused by too much acid, but by too little acid and by acid in the wrong place for too long. This can happen when the sphincter between the stomach and the esophagus relaxes, allowing the Mexican meal you just scarfed down to splash back up, making you feel like your heart is on fire. In many cases, heartburn and GERD can be caused by food intolerance, most commonly to dairy products.

Heartburn can be a once-in-a-while problem that is painful, but not serious, or it can be a regular plague that can cause severe health problems.

Heartburn is aggravated by alcohol, caffeine, chocolate and spicy and acidic foods, so if you suffer from occasional heartburn or long-term GERD, avoiding these foods will help. A low-carbohydrate diet will also be helpful, which is why your garden plays such an important role in relieving the pain and the disease.

Your Garden to the Rescue

Raw veggies including **lettuce, spinach, carrots** and **broccoli** are the best dietary solutions to heartburn because they are gentle and can help stop the inflammation caused by heartburn. Most doctors recommend lots of salads whether you have occasional heartburn or GERD. Avoid tomatoes and other acidic foods like citrus fruits since they tend to aggravate the condition.

Apples and **peaches** are soothing fruits as are **melons** and **pears**.

Don't turn to Prilosec! It can actually impair your digestive ability and make you dependent on the drug. Instead, you can get quick relief from several herbs, primarily from **fennel seeds** (just chew a teaspoon or so) that help relieve the spasms of the sphincter between the stomach and the esophagus.

The soothing effects of **chamomile** and **lemon balm** teas can also give you fast relief and relieve the inflammation caused by stomach acid where it doesn't belong.

I'm going to add in **ginger** here, although since it is tropical, you're unlikely to be able to grow it in your garden. It's a spice with enormous healing power, including helping calm the symptoms of heartburn and stopping the spasming of the sphincter. Make a tea of a one-inch piece of grated ginger root and find relief.

Again, you're unlikely to be growing **oats** and **wheat** in your garden (although you may decide this would be a fun experiment), but whole grains are a good source of selenium, which is study-proven to relieve GERD.

HEARING LOSS (*Also see Atherosclerosis*)

YOUR GARDEN RX: garlic, onions, echinacea, fenugreek, apples, dried beans, sunflower and pumpkin seeds

One-third of all people over 65 have some degree of hearing loss, most commonly caused by arterial plaque buildup in the small blood vessels of the inner ear or impaired nerve conductivity that blocks the transmission of sounds. Hearing loss can also be related to a buildup of earwax or long-term exposure to loud noises. Tinnitus (constant or intermittent ringing, buzzing or hissing noises) occurs in 85% of people with hearing loss.

Your Garden to the Rescue

Garlic, onions, apples and other foods that help lower cholesterol and reduce artery-clogging plaque may also help reduce hearing loss and a diet rich in these foods and low in saturated fats will almost certainly help prevent high cholesterol and arterial blockages.

A few droppersful of warm **garlic** or **fenugreek** infused olive oil will not only help soften impacted earwax, it may also neutralize microbial infection that can cause hearing loss.

Echinacea will help restore equilibrium and balance and control dizziness. It may also help prevent hearing loss due to infection and the buildup of scar tissue.

Tinnitus has been linked to niacin, zinc and magnesium shortfalls, so increase your intake of foods high in these nutrients, like **dried beans, pumpkin** and **sunflower seeds**.

HEART PROBLEMS

Heart disease, the number one killer in the Western world, is tragic because it is largely preventable. More people, both men and women (yes, women are just as vulnerable) die of heart disease than any other cause. About 770,000 Americans die every year of heart disease and strokes, more than from cancer and lung disease combined.

Yes, it's true that if your father and grandfather died of heart attacks, that increases your risk. But nothing increases your risk as much as the lifestyle choices you make in terms of diet and exercise. And if your risk is high because of heredity, it's even more important to do everything possible to protect your heart.

If you are obese or have diabetes, your risk of heart disease is huge. Since so many of us are obese *and* have diabetes, our collective risk for all sorts of heart disease is very high.

In general, a diet rich in antioxidant fruits and vegetables has time and again been proven to prevent heart disease and to help reverse the effects of heart disease once it begins, so virtually everything from your garden is good for you.

However, there are specific types of heart disease that can be helped by particular foods, so if you have any of the following conditions, please tailor your diet to address these problems.

ARRHYTHMIA (*Also see Heart Problems: Stroke Prevention*)

YOUR GARDEN RX: mustard and turnip greens, chili peppers, dried beans

Arrhythmia is sometimes called an "electrical storm of the heart." It sounds romantic, but it distinctly is not. Irregular heart rhythms, palpitations and atrial fibrillation all put you at high risk for a stroke.

Arrhythmia is often linked to a misfiring of the nerves that control the heartbeat. This can be caused by mineral imbalances.

Your Garden to the Rescue

Look for foods high in potassium and magnesium, such as **cantaloupe** and **mustard** and **turnip greens** and other **green leafy vegetables** to relax your heart muscle and help normalize your heartbeat.

Foods rich in B vitamins, including **dried beans** and **chili peppers**, will help with nerve conductivity for a steady heartbeat.

ATHEROSCLEROSIS (*Also see Heart Problems: Cholesterol*)

YOUR GARDEN RX: garlic, apples, blackberries, sunflower and pumpkin seeds, rosemary, purslane

Atherosclerosis, more commonly known as hardening of the

arteries, is actually a hardening and thickening of the arteries that supply the heart caused by fat and calcium deposits.

Atherosclerosis is conventionally treated with a battery of prescription drugs that all have a wide range of dangerous side effects, including heart failure. You've no doubt heard of the statin drugs that are supposed to lower cholesterol, which leaves fatty deposits that clog arteries. In fact, those same statin drugs actually impair your body's ability to make coenzyme Q10, an enzyme that, among many other things, reduces the accumulation of oxidized fats in blood vessels, eases high blood pressure and regulates the rhythm of the heart.

Your Garden to the Rescue

Garlic has been study-proven to help keep arteries clear and to lower cholesterol levels in people with high cholesterol. The quercetin in garlic is one of the most powerful antioxidants known and is directly linked to the reduction of artery-clogging fats.

High-fiber foods like **apples** can help lower cholesterol and reduce the fatty plaque that clogs arteries.

Vitamins C and E have been shown to stop the clumping of platelets of LDL ("bad") cholesterol in the arteries, so filling up on C-rich foods like **blackberries** and E-rich **pumpkin** and **sunflower seeds** can help.

Rosemary is another excellent antioxidant. In fact, it was once used to preserve meat—in other words, to prevent oxidation that leads to spoilage. That's what it does for your body, too!

The little-known vegetable **purslane** is the vegetable world's most potent source of blood-thinning omega-3 fatty acids, like those found in heart-healthy salmon, tuna and mackerel.

It's also the source of a perfectly balanced calcium-magnesium ratio.

Purslane leaves are also a good source of anti-inflammatory alpha-linolenic acid. Widely regarded as a weed, purslane is a leathery-leaved plant with bright pink flowers. It grows just about everywhere, so look for some at the edges of your yard, presuming you aren't using pesticides or herbicides on your lawn.

RX from Outside Your Garden

Pomegranate is an exceptionally high-ranking antioxidant that contains substances similar to ACE inhibitors, pharmaceuticals routinely used to treat atherosclerosis.

CHOLESTEROL (*Also see Heart Problems: Atherosclerosis*)

YOUR GARDEN RX: garlic, apples, dried beans, carrots, purslane

The liver manufactures and removes LDL cholesterol. The danger occurs when we eat a diet too high in saturated foods, unbalancing the body's natural cholesterol levels. High levels of total cholesterol, or high levels of LDL or "bad" cholesterol and/or blood fats called triglycerides, are all linked to atherosclerosis and heart attacks.

Cholesterol is a waxy substance that attaches itself to arteries, mainly the larger coronary arteries, and over time can completely block them. Pieces also can break loose and make their way to your heart, causing a heart attack, or to your brain, causing a stroke.

While cholesterol is naturally present in your body, manufactured by the liver, this HDL or "good" cholesterol actually helps usher "bad" cholesterol out of your body. A diet high in antioxidant foods will help raise HDL cholesterol.

Eating too much meat, cheese, butter, eggs and shellfish is likely to raise your LDL levels.

Your Garden to the Rescue

The more veggies you eat, the better. The same goes for fruits in somewhat more moderate levels (2–3 servings a day if you're not diabetic).

Garlic has been specifically proven to help lower total cholesterol levels as well as LDL cholesterol with it sulfur compounds like allicin, which quickly bonds with disease-causing free-radical oxygen molecules and ushers them out of your body.

Apples, with both soluble and insoluble fiber, and **dried beans**, with an abundance of fiber, help literally sweep those unhealthy fats from your system before they can enter your arteries and clog them up.

CONGESTIVE HEART FAILURE (*Also see Heart Problems: Arrhythmia*)

YOUR GARDEN RX: spinach, potatoes, dried beans, asparagus, beets, lettuce, tomatoes

Heart failure happens when your heart stops pumping efficiently. This causes blood to move through your body more slowly than normal and causes your heart to either stretch to try to pump more blood and more oxygen to your tissues or to become thickened and even less effective at beating.

Sometimes the kidneys are affected and fluid builds up in the tissues, causing fluid buildup in the lungs as well as weakness, dizziness and/or an irregular heartbeat.

Your Garden to the Rescue

Since magnesium is key to a strong and steady heartbeat, magnesium-rich foods like **spinach**, **potatoes** and **dried beans** may help strengthen your heart.

You'll also want to find some foods that are natural diuretics to help remove fluid from your body, like **asparagus** (which contains asparagine, an alkaloid that improves kidney function) and **beets**. The vitamin C in **tomatoes** helps the kidneys flush out toxins more efficiently. **Lettuce** improves metabolism and helps flush out excess fluids.

HEART ATTACK PREVENTION

YOUR GARDEN RX: tomatoes, cilantro, purslane, spinach, cantaloupe, hawthorn

If you are experiencing severe chest pain or any other signs of a heart attack, get to an emergency room immediately. This is where modern medicine excels. It just may save your life.

Heart attacks are caused by a sudden interruption in the blood to your heart, usually due to some type of obstruction in the artery, most often a clot or a piece of atherosclerotic plaque that has broken loose.

You don't have to be a medical expert to know the dangers of a heart attack. Many people do not survive and those who do usually have permanent damage to their hearts.

Your Garden to the Rescue

The lycopene in **tomatoes** has been study-proven to reduce the risk of heart attack dramatically, so keeping tomatoes, **watermelon** and **grapefruit** in your diet is a good preventive. All of these are good sources of lycopene.

After a heart attack, you'll want to do everything possible to strengthen your heart muscle and keep it strong with magnesium and potassium-rich foods, like **spinach** and **cantaloupe**. You'll also want to thin your blood with foods high in vitamin K, such as **cilantro**, and get a natural blood thinning dose of heart-healthy omega-3 fatty acids with **purslane**, a leafy weed-like vegetable.

Hawthorn leaves, flowers and berries act very much like many of the prescription drugs used to treat heart problems, including the ones that open blood vessels and reduce the stress placed on the heart.

RX from Outside Your Garden

Red wine is widely acknowledged as a good heart attack preventer, provided you drink it in moderation. For women this means a glass a day, and for men, not more than two glasses a day. This amount can reduce the risk of heart attack by half without increasing your risk of alcohol-related diseases.

HYPERTENSION (*High Blood Pressure*)

YOUR GARDEN RX: garlic, spinach, potatoes, onions, sunflower seeds, dried beans

Also known as high blood pressure, hypertension is a silent killer. Millions of Americans have it and don't know they have it, so they don't treat it, placing themselves at risk for heart attack and stroke.

If you have a blood pressure monitor or you make use of one at your local pharmacy, keep a few things in mind:

Blood pressure can change throughout the day. It's usually lowest early in the morning.

Blood pressure goes up when you're moving around. If you're taking a reading, sit still for at least five minutes before measuring it.

Blood pressure responds to stress and illness. When you visit your doctor's office, you may experience "white coat hypertension," which is one of the most common forms of elevated blood pressure but is usually temporary. If your doc tells you that your pressure is high, ask for a second reading later in the visit or ask if you can monitor your blood pressure at home over the coming month to determine whether there really is a problem. Many of us get nervous in the doctor's office and often blood pressure will be elevated anyway if you are there for some sort of illness. Long-term stress is another story that should be addressed to eliminate one of the most common underlying causes of hypertension.

Your target blood pressure reading should be 120/80. Anything higher could mean you have a problem. Anything significantly lower can indicate an adrenal insufficiency

Your Garden to the Rescue

Garlic is a primo vegetable to help relax blood vessels. Allicin, a sulfur compound that gives garlic its odor and its power, has been shown to relax blood vessels and lower blood pressure in addition to providing some other impressive heart-healthy benefits such as improving the body's ability to eliminate "bad" cholesterol, and normalizing heart rhythms.

Spinach, sunflower seeds and **dried beans** (think kidney beans, pintos and navy beans) are all good sources of magnesium. Your blood vessels are like rubber tubes that are stretched to the max, making them thin and taut. But if the tension on the tube is released, the tube becomes wider and more flexible. Magnesium works just like that in your arteries, helping blood flow more easily and lowering pressure.

Studies show that people who eat magnesium-rich diets have lower blood pressure.

Potatoes (baked or roasted, without butter or sour cream, please!) are an excellent source of potassium, which helps regulate fluid balance in the body. Excess water, fluid build-up, and bloating (usually caused by a sodium-potassium imbalance) put extra pressure on the blood vessels and increase blood pressure. Getting extra potassium from potatoes and the other foods mentioned in this section can help reduce the fluid buildup and normalize blood pressure.

PALPITATIONS

YOUR GARDEN RX: potatoes, spinach, walnuts, dried beans, red grapes, valerian

When your heart starts pounding like crazy, it could mean a number of things, but most likely it means you are stressed or have indulged in a little too much caffeine or alcohol. Palpitations that occur while you are in bed may accompany hot flashes for menopausal or perimenopausal women. Generally, unless you have a history of heart disease, palpitations are not cause for concern.

Your Garden to the Rescue

Foods high in magnesium and potassium will help regulate your heartbeat, so add more **potatoes, spinach, nuts** and **dried beans** to your diet. Grapes, and particularly **red grapes** are not only a great source of heart-healthy antioxidants, they are mineral rich and will give your heart the minerals it needs to function properly.

A few drops of valerian tincture can quickly calm a racing heart.

STROKE PREVENTION (*Also see Heart Problems: Heart Attack Prevention, Atherosclerosis*)

YOUR GARDEN RX: watermelon, spinach, broccoli, parsley

Strokes are often called "brain attacks" because most of them are caused by an obstruction of some sort that cuts off the blood supply to the brain, similar to the way a heart attack occurs when there is an obstruction of coronary blood vessels. However, about 15% of strokes are caused by burst blood vessels in the brain.

Atherosclerosis (hardening of the arteries) is a cause of stroke, with the carotid arteries in the neck being the most common place where blood flow is restricted.

The type of stroke caused by burst blood vessels is most often caused by uncontrolled high blood pressure.

Your Garden to the Rescue

Watermelon and other lycopene-rich foods like **tomatoes** and **papaya** are among the best possible hedges against stroke, since they are well known to protect against heart attacks. If you've had a stroke, opt for lots of raw foods, if you can chew them, or invest in a high-quality juicer to get as many fruits and vegetables into your system as possible.

Foods high in vitamin K, including all the dark green leafy vegetables—**broccoli, kale, collards, spinach** and **parsley**—will help thin out your blood and lower blood pressure.

Diuretic foods like **beets** and **lettuce** will also help keep your blood pressure under control.

HEMORRHOIDS

YOUR GARDEN RX: apples, dried beans, raspberries, chamomile, comfrey

Hemorrhoids are essentially varicose veins that occur inside your rectum or just around the anus. While they are usually not particularly a threat to your health, they certainly can be annoying with itching, bleeding and swelling, making sitting very uncomfortable.

Constipation and straining to produce a bowel movement cause these veins to rupture, as can pregnancy and labor.

You can prevent hemorrhoids by keeping your bowels healthy and avoiding constipation. If you already have hemorrhoids, preventing constipation is important so they can heal.

Your Garden to the Rescue

A high-fiber diet is the answer to preventing constipation and preventing irritation of existing hemorrhoids. All fruits and vegetables are good sources of fiber, so eat freely of your garden's bounty.

Pay special attention to getting enough fiber from sources, including **apples, dried beans** and **berries**, especially **raspberries**.

A gentle wash of chamomile tea can soothe the pain and itching, as can a homemade salve made from comfrey leaves.

HERPES

YOUR GARDEN RX: dried beans, bell peppers, broccoli, strawberries, cantaloupe

The herpes virus manifests in a number of ways, including the chickenpox that many of us experienced in childhood, cold sores, shingles and the sexually-transmitted genital herpes.

After the initial outbreak, the herpes virus remains dormant in your nervous system, sometimes for decades. It is known that people who had chickenpox as children are at risk for painful shingles later in life.

The trigger for shingles and genital herpes outbreaks is not fully understood, but stress is probably a factor in the reawakening of the virus, which then travels up the nerves to the skin, where it multiplies. People with compromised immune systems, such as are found in AIDS patients and those undergoing chemotherapy, are at higher risk for outbreaks.

Those who have genital herpes should never have sex with an uninfected person during an outbreak.

In recent years, a shingles vaccine has become available for people who had chickenpox as children. It has cut the expected outbreaks in half and may reduce the duration and intensity of those that do occur.

Your Garden to the Rescue

Eating foods rich in the amino acid lysine may shorten outbreaks. You'll find it in abundance in dried beans.

It is known that low vitamin C levels can put you at risk for an outbreak. Good sources of vitamin C like **bell peppers, strawberries, broccoli** and **cantaloupe** will help enhance your immune function and may prevent outbreaks.

HIATAL HERNIA (*Also see Heartburn*)

YOUR GARDEN RX: apples, all types of lettuce, celery, watermelon, cantaloupe

A hiatal hernia may produce many of the same symptoms as heartburn, but it is an entirely different problem. This condition occurs when the pyloric valve that separates the esophagus and the stomach becomes stretched, usually because of pregnancy or a large weight gain. It can also be caused by violent coughing, vomiting or straining with bowel movements. Smokers are at higher risk of hiatal hernia. In some cases, the hernia is present at birth.

The result is that part of the stomach actually pushes up through the diaphragm and into the esophagus.

About 50% of Americans over age 50 unknowingly have small hiatal hernias, but they have no symptoms. Large hiatal hernias may cause heartburn, belching, chest pain and nausea.

Conventional medicine treats hiatal hernia with acid reducers, the same ones used to treat heartburn. Occasionally, surgery is necessary to relieve the pain.

Heavy meals, alcohol, caffeine, smoking, chocolate, citrus fruits and tomato products tend to aggravate the condition, so most doctors recommend eating several small meals and avoiding trigger foods.

Your Garden to the Rescue

High-fiber fruits and vegetables, like apples, **lettuce, potatoes** with the skin and **celery** will ease the digestive process. You'll also need to drink a lot of water (but not with meals) and eat watery fruits like **watermelon** and **cantaloupe**.

HIVES (*Also see Allergies*)

YOUR GARDEN RX: chamomile, oregano, comfrey

Hives are itchy swollen patches on your skin that indicate an allergic reaction to something. The trick is figuring out what you're allergic to. It could be a medication, a food, jewelry, pets, insect bites, stress, a type of clothing or even a soap or laundry detergent.

Generally hives are more annoying than anything else, and, with luck, they fade within a few hours. But sometimes they signal a severe allergic reaction called anaphylaxis, which can be life threatening. If you get hives and have swelling around your mouth or eyes or if you have even the slightest difficulty swallowing, you need to get to an emergency room immediately because the swelling could cut off your ability to breathe.

However, your garden, more specifically your herb garden, can offer some relief for garden variety hives (pun intended!).

Your Garden to the Rescue

Oregano contains a range of natural anti-allergenics and antihistamines, so a salve or tea made from oregano as well as a few sprigs in your salad or pasta can really help.

Chamomile is the best "go to" herb to calm you down, and a cool wash of chamomile tea will also relieve the itching.

Comfrey salve is a personal favorite of mine. I use it for any kind of skin irritation.

RX from Outside Your Garden

A paste made of baking soda and water is wonderfully soothing.

HYPERACTIVITY (*Attention Deficit Hyperactivity Disorder or ADHD*)

YOUR GARDEN RX: pears, walnuts, pumpkin seeds, dried beans, potatoes, chamomile

ADHD or hyperactivity in children seems to have reached epidemic proportions. The exact causes are unknown, but there has been research that suggests that sugar, chemical additives and artificial colorings in processed foods may be a cause. Mineral imbalances, particularly an excess amount of copper and insufficient zinc, may also play role in hyperactivity.

Children usually grow out of this disorder by the time they are out of adolescence, but that time lag may seriously impair their education and consequently, their life prospects.

In the past twenty years or so since ADHD became widely known, parents have learned that restricting simple sugars from their children's diets is usually helpful.

Conventional medicine treats hyperactivity with a variety of anti-anxiety drugs, all of which have potentially serious side effects. Many parents believe that their children are unnecessarily medicated or are over-medicated.

Your Garden to the Rescue

Zinc-rich foods like **dried beans, pumpkin seeds** and **potatoes** eaten with the skins on are all helpful in correcting the copper–zinc imbalance that may be a factor in ADHD.

Pears, apples and other high-fiber foods can slow down the sugar excitability that often accompanies ADHD, but they should be eaten in moderation because they contain substantial amounts of natural sugars themselves.

Walnuts and other high-protein foods are also helpful in slowing the metabolism of simple sugars and potentially easing the hyperactivity symptoms.

RX from Outside Your Garden

Processed foods contain many chemicals and dyes that can aggravate or even cause ADHD. Adequate intake of omega-3 fatty acids is also critical to the treatment of ADHD.

HYPOTHYROIDISM (*Low Thyroid Function*)

YOUR GARDEN RX: strawberries, asparagus, garlic, spinach, pumpkin seeds, walnuts, pecans

Hypothyroidism means your thyroid gland is not producing enough hormones to properly regulate your metabolism.

Hypothyroidism has a dozen or more symptoms including fatigue, weight gain, dry hair, brittle fingernails, sensitivity to cold, absence of outer third of eyebrows, carpal tunnel syndrome, constipation and more. Low thyroid function has become increasingly common among perimenopausal women, with an estimated 30% or more having low thyroid function by the time they reach menopause.

Hypothyroidism is treated with replacement thyroid hormones. Although natural hormones have been in use for more than fifty years, doctors seem to be more reliant on synthetic thyroid hormone replacement, which can actually increase the symptoms that may have driven you to the doctor in the first place.

Since the thyroid is dependent on iodine to manufacture hormones, insufficient iodine intake can be an important factor in the disease.

Your Garden to the Rescue

Asparagus, strawberries, garlic and **spinach** are all excellent sources of thyroid-healthy iodine.

Pumpkin seeds are rich in tyrosine, an amino acid that combines with iodine to help your body make thyroid hormones.

Finally, selenium helps convert the plentiful T4 thyroid hormone thyroxine produced by your body into usable T3 (tri-iodothyronine), the more potent and usable form of thyroid hormones. Find it in abundance in all kinds of nuts, especially the **walnuts** or **pecans** you can grow in many parts of North America.

RX from Outside Your Garden

Celtic sea salt and most fish are excellent sources of iodine.

IMPOTENCE OR LOW LIBIDO

YOUR GARDEN RX: fava beans, garlic, pumpkin seeds, potatoes, turnip greens

Impotence and erectile dysfunction have received lots of attention in recent years because of the popularity of drugs that are supposed to take care of the problem. However, like most pharmaceuticals, the drugs intended to restore sexual function in men carry a price and can even lead to premature death from heart attack in men who were previously healthy.

While impotence was once thought to be mostly a psychological problem, medical science has identified physiological causes in the past couple of decades, most notably in men with diabetes who suffer from impaired circulation and nerve conductivity.

For any man, improving circulation to the small vessels that supply blood to the penis will help, as will improved nerve conductivity to improve sensation.

And yes, there are some men for whom impotence is psychological, so foods that induce relaxation and reduce anxiety can help.

Your Garden to the Rescue

If you need to relieve sexual anxiety, **fava beans** are among the best foods to help you produce more of the feel-good brain chemical dopamine. Want to really increase the dopamine? Sprout your fava beans to get ten times the dopamine as in plain dried beans.

Garlic helps open blood vessels and improves circulation to all parts of the body, including the small blood vessels that supply the penis.

Zinc-rich **pumpkin seeds and potatoes** are good source of the most important nutrient for sexual function. Those same pumpkin seeds are also good sources of vitamin E to help improve circulation.

Finally, good food sources of B vitamins will help improve nerve function and sensitivity. The fava beans and other dried beans, as well as potatoes, will give you more B.

INDIGESTION

YOUR GARDEN RX: celery, basil, peppermint, rosemary, fennel, chili peppers, radishes

Indigestion is an occasional fact of life for half of all Americans, and for 15 percent of us, it can happen daily. For many chronic sufferers, heartburn is the main symptom, but others experience bloating, belching, gas, nausea, vomiting, stomach rumbling and diarrhea.

Usually it is caused by simple overeating, a reaction to particular foods to which you may be sensitive, food poisoning, stress, or even a stomach ulcer.

If the indigestion is occasional, it will likely disappear on its own. If it is chronic, you'll need to take a careful look at your food consumption, the amounts you are eating and pinpoint foods that may be causing a reaction.

Your Garden to the Rescue

Radishes help calm an old-fashioned stomach ache and **peppermint** tea will soothe that churning feeling and relieve gas and bloating. **Basil**, another member of the mint family, is especially suited to gas relief.

Celery and **rosemary**, both widely prescribed in Europe to treat indigestion, contain dozens of painkillers, anti-inflammatories, anti-ulcer compounds and sedatives to ease your stomach and intestinal pain.

Chili peppers, contrary to the popular misconception that they trigger bellyaches and heartburn, actually help calm digestion and can even prevent ulcers.

Fennel seeds are a popular tummy soother in India after a satisfying spicy meal.

RX from Outside Your Garden

Ginger is a wonder food that is good for so many things. Its soothing compounds calm an irritated gut, relieve belching and nausea and help move food through the large and small intestines.

INFECTIONS

YOUR GARDEN RX: garlic, carrots, kale, strawberries, pumpkin seeds, echinacea

There are numerous types of infections, but all of them stem from a weakened immune system. While it is not possible to avoid infectious bacteria altogether (and we probably shouldn't), a strong immune system will fight off infection and minimize its effect, whether it is from a dirty cut or a yeast infection or a viral infection like a cold.

We all know the precautions, especially for colds and flu, but sometimes it is good to give your immune system a challenge that makes it stronger. Not that you should intentionally get an infection, but parents especially seem to be "germophobic" these days. Today's overabundance of antibacterial soaps and hand sanitizers and even countertop cleaners may actually be taking away the body's natural ability to build the immune system.

Your Garden to the Rescue

Garlic is an excellent source of the natural antibiotic quercetin, which has antiviral, antifungal and antibacterial benefits. Of course, eating garlic is the best way to boost your immune system whether or not you have in infection. You can also make a garlic poultice to draw out infection from a small wound.

Carrots are a good source of vitamin A to strengthen your immune system and vitamin C to notify it to start an attack against invaders, as are **collards, kale, spinach** and **strawberries.**

Add in a handful of **pumpkin seeds** for their zinc to boost your production of infection-fighting white blood cells and help you heal quickly.

INFERTILITY

YOUR GARDEN RX: pumpkin seeds, potatoes, dried beans, strawberries

In the modern world with all our stress and rushing from here to there, it's not surprising that infertility has become a problem for many couples.

On one hand, we're exhausted and disinclined to have sex or feel obligated to have it at the right time during the fertile periods. On the other hand, stress, smoking, excessive caffeine and alcohol consumption and poor diet make our bodies less likely to reproduce, either due to low sperm production in men or irregular ovulation in women.

We're also waiting later and later in life to start our families and science shows us that both sperm and eggs are less viable as we age.

Recent statistics indicate that at least 10 percent of couples in America who want to conceive are having difficulty.

Failure to ovulate is the main cause of women's infertility and may be caused by the hormonal fluctuations of peri-menopause, which has been identified in many women in their early 30s. Surgeries, miscarriages, infections and abdominal disease can also cause infertility.

For men, infertility is often caused by erectile dysfunction, which is closely linked to diabetes. Many men also have low sperm production or weak sperm that cannot perform the rigorous task of fertilizing an egg.

A diet that includes lots of antioxidant-rich fruits and vegetables will help both partners.

Your Garden to the Rescue

For both men and women, eating foods rich in vitamins C, E, and zinc have been shown to be helpful in overcoming infertility. **Strawberries** and all berries are very good sources of zinc and vitamin C, so they should be a regular part of your diet. Zinc deficiency has been especially identified in low sperm production in men. Low vitamin C levels have been found to slow sperm and cause them clump together.

Potatoes, dried beans and **pumpkin seeds** are also good sources of zinc and minerals.

RX from Outside Your Garden

If you want to get pregnant, both partners should abstain from smoking, caffeine and alcohol, since research shows that all of these contribute to infertility problems.

INSECT BITES

YOUR GARDEN RX: comfrey, plantain, pennyroyal

Insect bites have plagued humans and their four-legged friends since the beginning of time. Mosquito and gnat bites are generally annoying, but for the most part, they are not particularly dangerous. Some insect bites, however, can be dangerous, like those of ticks, bees, wasps, fire ants and certain kinds of spiders.

Your Garden to the Rescue

Prevention is the best remedy, but avoid toxic commercial bug sprays that contain DEET, which can cause neurological problems and even cardiac arrest.

You can also crush some **pennyroyal** and roll it up in a bandanna to wear around your neck or to tie onto your dog for effective insect repellent.

If you have been bitten, one of the quickest and most

effective remedies is to crush or better yet, chew a few **plantain** leaves and rub them on the site.

Comfrey is extremely helpful for more serious reactions. I dip a comfrey leaf briefly in boiling water and wrap it around the site, securing it with an old plastic bag or a piece of plastic wrap. The effects of all but the most serious bites will be gone in a few hours. I also make a salve of comfrey and eucalyptus to keep gnats and flies away and heal minor skin problems.

RX from Outside Your Garden

To make a great natural insect repellant, mix five drops of each of the following essential oils in a three-ounce spray bottle of water:

- Eucalyptus
- Lemongrass
- Pennyroyal
- Cedarwood
- Citronella

Apply liberally to yourself and your clothing. It's so effective, I use it on my horses and dogs as well.

INSOMNIA

YOUR GARDEN RX: sweet corn, dried beans, Swiss chard, pumpkin seeds, tart cherries, dill, chamomile, valerian

Insomnia affects most of us from time to time and, for about 30% of Americans, insomnia is a problem twice or more weekly.

A healthy diet, and especially avoidance of caffeine, are important to getting a good night's sleep, as is good "sleep hygiene," as the experts call it. This means preparing yourself for sleep by gradually winding down your day, avoiding stimulating music or television shows in the evening, perhaps taking a warm bath or drinking a soothing cup of **chamomile** tea.

One important part of sleep hygiene is to sleep in a room that is as dark as possible. That's because being the dark prompts your body to produce a hormone called melatonin, the regulator of your waking and sleeping cycles.

Your Garden to the Rescue

Melatonin-rich foods will help get your sleep cycle back into its natural rhythm. These include **sweet corn** and **tart cherries**.

If your insomnia is due to stress (who hasn't lain awake at night worrying about financial or health issues?), **dill** can help. It's the source of several brain chemicals that ease depression and anxiety, relax muscles, and soothe your nerves.

Nerve-soothing B vitamins, like those found in **dried beans**, can help you sleep.

Tryptophan, those brain chemicals that makes you sleepy after a big Thanksgiving turkey dinner, is a natural sleep inducer. How to grow it in your garden? Try **pumpkin seeds**.

Foods that contain good amounts of magnesium, like **Swiss chard** and **potatoes**, help you sleep because low magnesium can cause your brain to become overstimulated, robbing you of sleep.

Valerian, even though it smells like dirty socks (or worse), is a powerful sleep aid that should be used sparingly. It can have effects similar to those of sleeping pills.

IRRITABLE BOWEL SYNDROME

YOUR GARDEN RX: apples, blueberries, winter squash, spinach, peppermint, fennel, sage

Irritable bowel syndrome is a perplexing and painful basket of symptoms that can range from constipation to diarrhea (often both) and is often characterized by severe gas, bloating and abdominal cramps.

Since flare-ups can usually be separated into diarrhea-related attacks or constipation-dominant ones, the foods you use to help control IBS will be dependent on which type you are experiencing.

Although the cause of IBS is not entirely understood, it is known that certain things can cause a flare-up, especially such as eating a high-fat meal or simply eating a very large meal.

Your Garden to the Rescue

If you have the abdominal cramps, bloating and gas typical of both phases of IBS, it is common sense to avoid dried beans and other gas-producing vegetables like broccoli, cabbage and cucumbers. **Peppermint, fennel** and **sage**—better yet, all of them together in an admittedly strange-tasting tea—are excellent carminatives (anti-gas herbs). Peppermint is also a good stomach soother and relieves cramps.

If you are suffering from a constipation flare-up, look for foods that contain a lot of fiber for a gentle natural laxative effect, like **apples, blueberries, spinach** and **winter squash,** especially **acorn** and **butternut.** A salad of early spring greens like **spinach, Swiss chard** and **beet greens** makes an excellent source of fiber and good omega-3 fats to help your bowels get moving.

Apples are a good food for IBS sufferers because they can work both ways, as a natural laxative or to stop diarrhea, bringing your colon back into balance. Look to high-fiber foods to help relieve the diarrhea, too.

JOINT PAIN (*Also see Arthritis*)

YOUR GARDEN RX: chili peppers, oregano, spinach, cantaloupe, broccoli

Joint pain is almost always caused by some sort of inflammation of the joints, usually due to wear and tear over the years that causes deterioration of the cartilage, a soft tissue cushion that separates the bones. However, joint pain can be caused by an injury or, in the case of rheumatoid arthritis, by an immune system overreaction to your body's own cartilage. Over time, joint pain can reduce mobility and negatively affect quality of life.

Inflammatory compounds in highly acidic meats (beef and pork primarily) may aggravate the inflammation, so if you're suffering from joint pain, you might consider cutting back on your red meat intake.

For some people, the pain may be caused by an allergic-type reaction to certain kinds of foods. Dairy foods are the most frequent culprits in this type of joint pain, so eliminating them may help. Increasing your water consumption may also help.

Knees, hips and hands are the most common sites of joint pain, although it can occur anywhere. If you are overweight, losing weight can ease the strain on your joints.

Conventional medical treatment for joint pain is most often NSAIDS (non-steroidal anti-inflammatory drugs), a class of prescription and nonprescription drugs (like aspirin, acetaminophen, and ibuprofen) that can cause serious problems ranging from gastrointestinal bleeding to heart attacks and liver failure.

Your Garden to the Rescue

Capsaicin, a compound found in **chili peppers**, helps reduce pain and inflammation. Eating hot chilies and using a salve or cream made from them (or cayenne pepper) can give you relief. The multifunctional beauty of chilies is they also contain salicylates that act like aspirin to relieve pain.

Foods high in vitamin C can help rebuild collagen, the building block of cartilage. Look for your vitamin C in **spinach, cantaloupe, broccoli** and **berries**.

Oregano is another excellent anti-inflammatory, with dozens of ingredients that help relieve swelling and pain.

RX from Outside Your Garden

Ginger, turmeric and holy basil (an Indian herb, not the same as our garden basil) have some of the most powerful anti-inflammatory compounds known and they're free of side effects.

KIDNEY STONES

YOUR GARDEN RX: blueberries, radishes, potatoes, cantaloupe, dried beans

Kidney stones are the result of crystal formation of certain minerals in urine, particularly calcium salts. These minerals actually form tiny rough stones in the kidneys that the body eventually attempts to pass through the ureters (tiny urinary tubes), causing an interruption of urinary flow and intense pain in the lower back, sides and pelvic area. Kidney stones occur most often in men over 50. Conventional medicine has, in recent years, developed a nonsurgical shock wave treatment that dissolves larger stones. Increased water intake is key to the treatment of kidney stones to help flush the kidneys and make the urine less acidic.

Your Garden to the Rescue

Blueberries and **radishes** are well-known diuretics that can help flush the kidneys and help usher out excess mineral deposits. Drinking lots of tea made from **dandelion** leaves and roots can help prevent the formation of kidney stones. **Cantaloupes** and other juicy fruits like peaches and grapes can help increase your hydration levels. **Potatoes**, high in potassium, can help prevent kidney stones since many kidney stone sufferers have low potassium levels. **Dried beans**, a good source of magnesium, can help regulate blood calcium and prevent the formation of stones.

RX from Outside Your Garden

Cranberries and cranberry juice are known to be very helpful in addressing and preventing kidney stones and other urinary problems.

LEG PAIN (Leg Cramps, Restless Leg Syndrome, Intermittent Claudication)

YOUR GARDEN RX: garlic, onions, broccoli, cauliflower, tomatoes, sweet potatoes, sunflower seeds, red grapes, dried beans, pumpkin, blueberries

There are several types of leg pain, ranging from cramps to restless leg syndrome, which can rob you of sleep, to serious conditions like intermittent claudication, a circulatory problem that can be extremely painful and potentially disabling.

Your Garden to the Rescue

Simple muscle cramps (sometimes we call them Charley horses) usually happen when your leg has been in one place for some time and you move it suddenly, causing the muscle to rebel and spasm. Usually the pain subsides in a minute or two with a little stretching and massage. However, if muscle cramps are a common occurrence, you may need more calcium and magnesium in your diet to help your muscles contract and relax properly. **Broccoli, tomatoes** (better yet, tomato juice), **sweet potatoes** and **sunflower seeds** are good sources of essential magnesium and potassium that will help prevent leg cramps.

Iron deficiency is a contributor to restless leg syndrome, so if you've experienced that can't-sit-or-lie-still feeling, look at your iron intake and see if it is lacking. While red meat is the best source of iron, you can get moderate amounts in **dried beans**, especially **kidney beans**, and **pumpkin**.

Intermittent claudication with severe cramping and tingling in thighs, buttocks, and legs is a form of peripheral artery disease (PAD) that can be serious. It is caused by clogged blood vessels in the legs and puts you at risk of a heart attack. People with PAD often experience great pain even when they try walking a short distance. Because PAD is a heart disease, following the guidelines for cholesterol, blood pressure and other heart-related problems is helpful.

Red grapes and **blueberries** are among the most powerful antioxidants and will promote heart health. **Garlic** and **onions** are also antioxidants with special properties that make blood less likely to clot.

LIVER DISEASE

YOUR GARDEN RX: apples, onions, green beans, grapes, broccoli,
   dried beans, spinach, milk thistle

Liver disease is a serious problem that can have a variety of causes, primarily including hepatitis B (liver cancer), alcoholism (cirrhosis) and obesity (fatty liver disease). Since the liver is the organ that cleanses the body of toxins, stores fat-soluble vitamins and manufactures amino acids and cholesterol, any disease that affects the liver has far-ranging and serious consequences.

However, the liver has a unique ability among the body's organs: It can function even if only 25% of it is healthy enough and the damaged cells can be regenerated.

Your Garden to the Rescue

Flavonoids, nature's warrior antioxidants, can be particularly helpful in fighting liver disease. In European countries, silymarin, a particular flavonoid found in **milk thistle**, actually saved the lives of many people with cirrhosis.

Other flavonoid-rich foods that promote liver health include **onions, green beans, grapes, broccoli, celery** and **spinach**.

Dried beans and **leafy greens** are also good sources of omega-3 fatty acids that promote good liver function, and the dried beans are also good sources of protein.

LUPUS

YOUR GARDEN RX: broccoli, cabbage, pumpkin seeds, sunflower seeds,
   borage

Systemic lupus erythematosus, commonly called lupus, is an autoimmune disease that has many arthritis-like symptoms, including severe joint pain.

Its cause is unknown, although there is speculation that lupus may be caused by a virus. For many people, lupus is a manageable disease, but in severe cases, it can cause organ failure, usually starting with the kidneys. In those cases, it is life threatening.

Among the many symptoms of lupus is extreme sensitivity to sunlight, so many people with the disease are deficient in vitamin D, a hormone-like vitamin that the body manufactures through exposure to sunlight.

Since people with lupus tend to have high cholesterol levels, you might want to look at the Heart Disease entry.

Some foods may increase the intensity of the symptoms of lupus. It's usually best to avoid foods that have alfalfa in any form. Also, for many people, mushrooms and some smoked foods may cause problems.

Lupus is often treated with NSAIDS (non-steroidal anti-inflammatory drugs), but in severe cases, steroids are necessary to control the pain. While there is no cure for this potentially deadly disease, lifestyle and medical management can often control it.

Your Garden to the Rescue

Flavonoid-rich cruciferous vegetables like **broccoli** and **cabbage** contain substances called indoles that are helpful in cleansing the body of harmful types of estrogen, a concern since most lupus sufferers are women.

Pumpkin and **sunflower seeds** are good sources of vitamin E, zinc and selenium, all-important to people with lupus to help them fight inflammation.

Borage and evening primrose are important sources of gamma linolenic acid (GLA), unique fatty acids that balance the acidic and inflammatory acids we encounter when we eat meat.

MENOPAUSE AND PERIMENOPAUSE

YOUR GARDEN RX: black beans, celery, dill, fennel, walnuts

Hormone fluctuations begin long before a woman stops menstruating. Some women start experiencing perimenopause, which is when estrogen and progesterone start leapfrogging, as early as their mid-thirties.

When a woman enters menopause, it means she no longer has menstrual periods (medically defined as having no periods for 12 months) and is no longer able to become pregnant. Postmenopausal women have a greater risk of heart attack and stroke because they have lost the protective effects of estrogen. Bones may also become more brittle at this stage of life, necessitating mineral supplementation to prevent osteoporosis.

Perimenopause carries with it a laundry list of unpleasant symptoms, including hot flashes, night sweats, mood swings, depression, memory loss, joint pain and weight gain.

Your Garden to the Rescue

Black beans and other **dried beans** are a good source of plant estrogens (saponins, phytosterols, isoflavones and lignans) without some of the potential estrogenic excesses of soy and they may actually help protect you against estrogen-related cancers like breast cancer.

Celery, dill and fennel, all of which are in the same plant family, have mild and gentle estrogenic compounds to relieve symptoms like hot flashes and give you long-term protection against heart disease and cancer.

Walnuts are an excellent source of omega-3 fatty acids that can help preserve memory, lessen mood swings and ease depression and hot flashes.

When perimenopause is over and you are officially menopausal or postmenopausal, you'll want to follow all the guidelines to protect your heart and bones and prevent cancer. You may continue to experience some of the symptoms of menopause for several years. A diet rich in all kinds of garden goodies will help keep you healthy for years to come.

RX from Outside Your Garden

The soy controversy: Some experts think soy will naturally help replace lost estrogen and others think it is harmful. There's not much doubt that soy will relieve hot flashes, but there are other less risky means of addressing this symptom such as supplements made from black cohosh, chasteberry or wild yam.

MENSTRUAL DISORDERS AND PMS

YOUR GARDEN RX: dried beans, walnuts, sweet potatoes, apples, carrots, tomatoes, strawberries, cantaloupe, parsley

Menstrual "inconveniences" are common. Most women experience some problems, either before their periods or during them: cramping, breast tenderness, constipation or diarrhea, mood swings, irritability, bloating, headaches and food cravings. This is generally known as PMS (premenstrual syndrome). Its basket of symptoms can be a minor annoyance or a major life challenge, depending on its severity.

Research shows that women who exercise several times a week are less likely to have PMS. PMS is also less prevalent in women who engage in healthy eating habits, avoiding processed foods, caffeine and alcohol in the days leading up to their periods.

Conventional medicine doesn't have much to offer women who suffer from severe menstrual problems except NSAIDS like ibuprofen, which may be moderately effective, and anti-depressants, which aren't very effective in their own right.

Your Garden to the Rescue

B vitamins go a long way toward soothing jangled nerves, so increase your intake of B-rich **dried beans** and **sweet potatoes** in the days before your period begins to keep your mood on a more even keel.

Walnuts are a great source of magnesium to ease mood swings and cramping, plus they are a good source of pain and inflammation-relieving omega-3 fatty acids. **Broccoli, kale** and other cruciferous vegetables are also helpful against cramps because of their muscle-relaxing calcium content.

Even a tablespoon or two of fresh **parsley** will help ease bloating, and fiber-dense, moderately sweet **apples** and **carrots** can quell the sugar cravings if you give them twenty minutes or so to take effect.

If you have unusually heavy periods, you are at risk for anemia, so increasing your iron intake is a good idea. Since you don't want to "beef up" too much with red meat (which remains the best source of iron), look for iron-rich veggies like spinach (remember Popeye the Sailor Man?), pumpkin seeds and dried beans. **Tomatoes, strawberries, cantaloupe** and other good sources of vitamin C will help you absorb the iron better.

MUSCLE CRAMPS (*Also see Leg Pain*)

YOUR GARDEN RX: spinach, potatoes, dried beans, sweet potatoes, beet greens, tomatoes, spinach.

Muscle cramps are caused by a muscle that contracts and then doesn't relax or goes into a spasm, contracting and relaxing rapidly. If you've ever felt the pain of a Charley horse, you don't forget it soon.

While calf muscles most often suffer Charley horses, any muscles can cramp. It's common to have cramps in feet, hands and back muscles.

Muscle cramps are more common in hot weather. Since dehydration is one cause of muscle cramping, inadequate water intake in the summer probably contributes to the cramping.

Muscles can't move unless they receive a message from the brain and minerals are the carriers of those messages. If you have a shortfall of any of the electrolyte minerals— calcium, potassium, sodium or magnesium—your muscles are more likely to cramp. While all these minerals are important to muscle contraction, magnesium is the controller, so a shortfall of magnesium can keep the others from being absorbed.

Your Garden to the Rescue

Clearly, magnesium-rich foods like **potatoes** with the skins on and **dried beans**, especially black-eyed peas and kidney and pinto beans, are a big part of the answer to muscle cramps.

Potatoes are a great bet here, because they are also an excellent source of cramp-relieving potassium, as are **sweet potatoes, beet greens** and **tomatoes**.

Leafy greens, including **spinach** and **collards**, are good sources of potassium as well, and they are also rich in calcium for added relief from involuntary muscle contractions.

NAIL PROBLEMS

YOUR GARDEN RX: dried beans, broccoli, peas, spinach, raspberries, cantaloupe, tomatoes, celery, garlic, chamomile

Nails are a barometer of your overall health. Although you may sometimes nervously pick at your fingernails or bite them, brittle, breaking and thin nails are most often indicators of a nutrient deficiency. They also can be a symptom of certain types of anemia or hypothyroidism. (See the entries about these conditions for more information.) In addition, some nail problems are caused by fungal infections.

To be strong, your nails need a steady supply of high-quality protein. Like every other part of your body, they are also dependent on adequate water to remain moist.

Weak and brittle nails can also be caused by our affection for manicures and pedicures. The harsh chemicals in polish removers and the formaldehyde in many nail polishes can damage nails. Artificial nails can cause severe damage to the nails and further weaken them by making them susceptible to fungal infection.

Your Garden to the Rescue

Dried beans are among the best vegetable sources of iron, so include some in your diet daily if you want to improve your nail health. **Broccoli, peas** and **spinach** are also good sources of iron.

You'll want to add foods high in vitamin C to help your body absorb the iron: **raspberries, cantaloupe** and **tomatoes**.

If your problems are caused by a fungal infection, eating celery and garlic can help your system fight off the infection. If you are bold enough, you can also make a poultice of mashed **garlic** or a wash of **chamomile** tea, since chamomile has more than two dozen antiseptic compounds.

NAUSEA

YOUR GARDEN RX: peppermint, sage, fennel, cilantro, rosemary, oregano, potatoes

Nausea can have a number of causes, ranging from simple indigestion to pregnancy-related morning sickness, motion sickness, headaches and even food poisoning.

Most people have no interest whatever in eating when they are nauseated, although in some cases, dry toast or a little bit of rice may help calm the queasies. Sometimes the easiest way is to go ahead and vomit and get it over with, even if you have an aversion to the loss of control that accompanies vomiting.

Be sure to drink as much water as you can comfortably get down when you're feeling queasy to avoid dehydration, but it is absolutely fine to listen to your body skip eating for a day or even two unless you have diabetes. Water intake is especially important if you have a tummy bug that is also giving you diarrhea.

Your Garden to the Rescue

If you feel at all like eating, go with something very mild and bland, like a plain baked **potato**. While some people think dairy foods are a good idea, milk or cottage cheese can actually worsen the problem if you're queasy.

Turn to your herb garden for the best answers and the quickest relief. Concoct a tea containing as many of the following herbs as you like:

Peppermint, for general digestive calming

Oregano, for its sedative and pain-relieving properties

Cilantro or **coriander** and **chamomile**, which can actually help you vomit if that is what you need

Fennel, famous in India for its indigestion relief

Raspberry leaf, which is so safe it is widely recommended for morning sickness

Sage and **rosemary**, for their stomach-calming properties as well as helping to ease the anxiety that often accompanies nausea

NERVE PAIN *(Also see Herpes)*

YOUR GARDEN RX: spinach, potatoes, melon, sunflower seeds, pumpkin seeds

Nerve pain can have a number of causes:

- An accident may have damaged or constricted nerves, causing them to either send unceasing pain signals or to become numb.

- Shingles and other herpes outbreaks are caused by the herpes virus, often acquired if you had chickenpox as a child or contracted genital herpes as an adult. It remains dormant in the nervous system until a flare up occurs through the nerves, often decades later.

- Sciatica is a type of nerve pain primarily caused by degenerating discs in the lower back.

- Diabetes can cause peripheral neuropathy, a numbing of the nerves usually in the feet, that leads to more amputations that any other non-accident-related cause.

- Many medications, including those used for chemotherapy, can cause nerve damage.

- Nutritional deficiencies, most often of vitamin B12, can cause weakness or burning sensations.

- There are also a number of diseases, like Lou Gehrig's disease (amyotrophic lateral sclerosis) and trigeminal neuralgia, which affect the nerves.

Your Garden to the Rescue

Nerves are directly affected by B-complex vitamins, so look for B-rich foods like **spinach, potatoes** and **melons** to help ease nerve pain. Note: One of the best nerve-pain relievers is vitamin B12, found only in animal products.

Vitamin E shortfalls can also cause a form of neuralgia, so be sure you're getting enough E with **sunflower** and **pumpkin seeds**.

OBESITY/WEIGHT CONTROL

YOUR GARDEN RX: potatoes, turnips, apples, dried beans, grapes, chili peppers

If you've been trying to control your weight, you know very well that it's an incredibly complex task. Doctors and other so-called experts will tell you that you need to eat less and exercise more. They'll also tell you that it is "calories in/calories burned"—a mathematical equation. It's not that simple.

Each individual's biological makeup is unique. That's why your best friend (especially if he's male) can annoyingly skip lunch and lose five pounds while you eat like a bird for weeks and the scale doesn't budge a bit. Your weight depends on a broad spectrum of variables, including your body type, metabolic rate, heredity, amount of body fat and, of course, caloric intake. Yes, calories do play a part—but they are not the whole story.

I wish I could give you more encouragement, but the best advice is to get to know your own body. It's surprising how many of us do not. The basics are no-brainers:

- Eat when you're hungry.
- Stop eating when you are full.
- Don't eat when you're not hungry.
- Especially don't eat when you are stressed.
- Avoid multitasking when you eat to prevent overeating.
- Chew your food carefully.
- Drink lots of water, but not with meals.
- And perhaps most important, enjoy your food!

Your Garden to the Rescue

You can freely eat virtually all fruits and vegetables when you are trying to control your weight. You may be surprised to learn that includes **potatoes**, an underrated vegetable with a multitude of health benefits. Among them, potatoes help you feel full longer, helping you avoid the temptations of less healthful foods. Other starchy root vegetables like **turnips** and **rutabagas** have the same effect. Of course, as always, it's best to forego the butter and sour cream. Salsa makes a healthy diet-friendly topping for baked potatoes.

Apples are another "high satisfaction" food, low on the glycemic index, low in calories and full of appetite-satisfying fiber and pectin.

All **dried beans** are high in fiber, low in fat, low in calories and packed with health benefits, so they're among the best foods you can adopt for weight control.

The same goes for all kinds of hot peppers: they're nutrient dense, low in calories, non-existent on the fat scale, and their "heat" helps rev up your metabolism. Try adding a little hot sauce to that salsa on your baked potato.

OSTEOPOROSIS (*Also see Bone Loss*)

YOUR GARDEN RX: blackberries, broccoli, cauliflower, dried beans, kale

Osteoporosis is a loss of bone density over time, usually affecting the elderly and most often postmenopausal women. The first sign of osteoporosis is usually a loss of height due to the weakening of the spine caused by bone loss. Bone pain, tenderness, fractures with little or no trauma and back and neck pain due to fractures of spinal bones are common.

The primary cause of osteoporosis is low estrogen levels in women after menopause. It can also be caused by smoking, excessive alcohol consumption, rheumatoid arthritis, chronic kidney disease, hyperparathyroidism, eating disorders and the long-term use of corticosteroid medications like prednisone and methylprednisolone.

Conventional medicine mainly treats osteoporosis with a class of drugs called bisphosphonates, which attach themselves to calcium molecules in the bones and slow the breakdown of bone tissue. The biggest concern with these drugs has been that they can actually cause splintering types of fractures that are exceptionally difficult to treat and they've specifically been associated with deterioration of the jaw-bone.

Your Garden to the Rescue

Opt for garden produce that gives you a wide variety of minerals essential to bone health, including magnesium, manganese, copper, phosphorous and potassium. **Blackberries** are excellent sources of many different minerals, so add them to your diet on a daily basis, if possible. **Broccoli, cauliflower, kale, cabbage** and **collards** are also not only good sources of calcium, they are good sources of all the minerals you need for strong bones.

Dried beans are among our best vegetable sources of protein, an important building block for strengthening bones and important to the production of hormones that help build bone tissue.

PAIN RELIEF (Also see Arthritis, Back Pain, Joint Pain, Headache, Nerve Pain)

YOUR GARDEN RX: chili peppers, oregano, peppermint

Pain is a very subjective thing that can come from many sources and have many causes. Even though none of us like pain, it actually is your friend and lets you know when something is wrong. Imagine the consequences if you didn't feel pain when you put your hand on a hot stove.

Pain signals are carried along nerve pathways to the brain. The brain interprets the pain and takes action, if necessary, such as pulling your hand back from the hot stove or putting your hand on your jaw if you have a toothache.

But we all know that pain can be much more than a minor inconvenience. It can disrupt our lives, whether it's a simple toothache or something really serious. Chronic pain can certainly have life-altering effects.

Conventional medicine treats long-term pain with increasingly addictive painkillers and sometimes with antidepressants and anti-anxiety drugs as well.

Your Garden to the Rescue

Capsaicin, the primary ingredient in **hot peppers**, is one of nature's most powerful pain relievers precisely because it blocks those pain signals to the brain using "Substance P," a pain-relieving element of capsaicin that science hasn't yet entirely defined. But science does know that it works for pain signals that travel along the nerves. It won't work for the pain of a strained muscle.

You can make a capsaicin cream by adding finely chopped chilies to your favorite hand cream. When you apply it, your skin must be completely dry or you'll get a burning sensation that will be its own pain. Be sure to carefully wash your hands after applying the capsaicin cream.

You also can chop the chilies into a soup, stew, or salad or just add a few drops of hot sauce to your favorite foods.

Oregano is a literal soup of painkillers, as is **peppermint**, so drinking them as a tea or making a salve from them can give you relief.

RX from Outside Your Garden

Ginger is one of the most potent anti-inflammatories known, so a tea or even a ginger salve can relieve pain effectively. With its dozens of healing ingredients, it's a good idea to keep ginger on hand at all times.

PNEUMONIA

YOUR GARDEN RX: blueberry, spinach, sweet potatoes, garlic, elderberry, onion, celery, oregano, rosemary, basil

Pneumonia is most often the result of a challenged immune system. That means it rarely occurs by itself but comes in the aftermath of an immune system challenge like a cold, flu, bronchitis or a hospital-acquired infection.

Pneumonia can be life threatening and is tricky to treat because it can be caused by a virus or by bacteria with the added complication that many modern pneumonia strains are antibiotic resistant. Infrequently, pneumonia can be caused by a fungal infection.

Conventional medicine usually treats pneumonia with antibiotics, which will be ineffective if the cause is viral or fungal and only moderately effective if it is bacterial.

Your Garden to the Rescue

Prevention is your best defense against pneumonia, so any vegetables, fruit, or herbs that boost your immune system will serve you well. These include antioxidant-rich **blueberries, sweet potatoes, spinach** and citrus fruits if you can grow them. Preventing colds and flu or treating them at the outset is the second prong in our approach to pneumonia prevention. Garlic is a star here again because of its antimicrobial properties, meaning it can fight viral, bacterial and fungal infections. **Onions, elderberries, celery, oregano, rosemary** and **basil** also carry those antimicrobial properties. A general diet rich in these foods will help prevent colds and flu, and increasing your intake at the first sign of these illnesses will help prevent pneumonia.

Pneumonia can potentially be life threatening, so see your

health care practitioner at the first signs, which include difficulty breathing, mild to high fever, shaking chills and/or severe cough, sometimes with green, yellow or bloody mucus.

ROSACEA (*Also see Acne*)

YOUR GARDEN RX: cherries, blackberries, blueberries, comfrey

Rosacea is a skin condition similar to acne, without the characteristic blackheads you'd find with acne.

Most information about rosacea and food contains warnings to avoid hot, spicy foods that increase blood flow to the face. Many sources also recommend limiting alcohol, sugar, caffeine and animal fats. Not coincidentally, most of these rosacea triggers are acidic foods and there is a school of thought that alkalizing your diet will also help relieve the condition.

Your Garden to the Rescue

Cherries, blackberries and **blueberries** help constrict swollen and inflamed blood vessels, including those tiny ones that make your face red.

Comfrey, used as a salve or cream or even as a wash, can also help constrict those inflamed blood vessels and reduce redness. It is not advisable to use comfrey as a tea because there are some reports it can be toxic to the liver.

SINUSITIS (*Also see Allergies*)

YOUR GARDEN RX: chili peppers, bell peppers, garlic, onions, oregano

Sinusitis is an infection in the sinuses, those hollow cavities around your face to which we rarely pay attention until they fill up with mucus and cause pressure, headaches, postnasal drip, cough and general misery.

Sinusitis generally follows a cold and can be caused by viruses, bacteria, fungi or all three. Usually the infection clears up on its own in four to six weeks, but those weeks can feel very long indeed with the misery of sinusitis.

Sinusitis can also be triggered by allergies, most often to cigarette smoke, but some food allergies can also trigger the immune reaction.

Conventional medicine usually treats sinusitis with antibiotics, which may be effective if the infection is bacterial, but will be completely ineffective if it is viral or fungal. Nasal sprays are also often used, but these can become habit forming.

Your Garden to the Rescue

The congestion is caused by the formation of histamines, chemical compounds your body produces when you're having an allergic reaction. **Garlic** and **onions** are the best sources of quercetin, a compound that acts like an antihistamine and also helps reduce inflammation.

Bell peppers and other food sources of vitamin C boost your immune system and offer the added benefit of natural defense against viral infections.

Oregano is an excellent natural antihistamine and offers bonus antiseptic and antioxidant benefits, so think about a vitamin C–rich **tomato** sauce heavily spiced with oregano when you have sinus problems.

RX from Outside Your Garden

Washing your sinuses with warm, filtered water with a little sea salt added is one of the best ways to treat sinusitis and to prevent its return. Use sea salt to prevent irritation and either slowly "drink" the water through your nose from a glass, spitting it out your mouth, or use one of those handy neti pots designed just for this purpose.

SMOKING CESSATION (*Also see Appetite Control, Obesity/Weight Control*)

YOUR GARDEN RX: apples, celery, broccoli, strawberries, cherries, tomatoes, pumpkin

If you're a smoker, you've heard it over and over again: You *must* stop before you do irreparable damage to your health. Some say it is more difficult to stop smoking than to beat a heroin addiction, so use whatever tools you have, even prescription drugs, to overcome this deadly addiction. Ask your doctor for help.

Yes, it will be difficult, but it is also the most positive thing you can do for yourself and those you love. Having a buddy along the way will help, as will participating in one of the many support groups in every city and town.

Many people who smoke are worried that they will gain weight when they quit and it's true, there is an association between stopping smoking and gaining weight. Look for foods that help stop cravings—not only for cigarettes, but also for food.

Your Garden to the Rescue

Look for foods known to help stop cravings, primarily **apples** and **celery**, both of which contain anti-craving substances.

According to an interesting study from Duke University, smokers reported that eating fruits and vegetables made their cigarettes taste worse. That may be why smokers eat far fewer fruits and vegetables than do non-smokers.

You'll also want to increase your intake of foods that protect you from the free-radical damage associated with cigarette smoking. **Broccoli** and other cruciferous vegetables are among the best at this, providing several excellent anti-cancer compounds, including sulphoraphane.

Cherries and **strawberries** contain a unique phytochemical, ellagic acid, which neutralizes hydrocarbons, especially the cancer-causing chemicals in tobacco smoke.

Tomatoes and other pink and red-colored fruits offer antioxidant protection through a carotenoid called lycopene, which has been shown to offer more cancer protection than most other fruits and vegetables.

Pumpkin and other orange or yellow veggies and fruits may protect against cancers most commonly attributed to smokers—lung, colon, skin, and kidney—because of their high levels of beta carotene.

RX from Outside Your Garden

Stop cravings with the amino acid l-glutamine. Just break open a capsule and sprinkle its tasteless contents on your tongue. L-glutamine can banish even the strongest cravings for cigarettes and is even effective for drug addictions.

SPRAINS (*Also see Pain Relief*)

YOUR GARDEN RX: cabbage, parsley, calendula, arnica

A bad sprain may take longer to heal than a broken bone because the injury to soft tissue, ligament and muscles can be slow to heal.

Sprains involve stretching or tearing of the ligaments and muscles. The most common sprain site is the ankle. If the ligament is ruptured (you may hear a loud popping sound when this occurs), surgery may be necessary.

Conventional medicine also wisely recommends keeping the inflamed area cool with ice, elevating it to the level of the heart and avoiding using the affected area as much as possible.

Your Garden to the Rescue

The advice of conventional medicine is sound, but you may be able to speed the healing with a poultice made of **cabbage** leaves or **parsley**, both folk remedies that help reduce swelling and ease the pain. Parsley has the added benefit of increasing circulation in the injured area and speeding healing.

Calendula (a marigold-like flower easily grown in most North American gardens) and **arnica** (a daisy-like flower found mostly in the Western states) both have anti-inflammatory properties and are best used in a salve or cream.

STRESS

YOUR GARDEN RX: potatoes, celery, green beans, borage, lavender, chamomile

It's impossible to avoid stress in this modern world. From the moment we get up in the morning, whether we flip on the radio for the morning news or wrangle kids into their school clothes while preparing lunches and getting dressed for work, for most of us the day begins with stress-inducing situations and ends the same way as, exhausted, we fall into bed. Often the stress doesn't even end at bedtime as we toss and turn, unable to sleep because of the to-do lists running through our minds, then we waken the next morning short on sleep to start the stress cycle all over again.

When we are stressed, our adrenal glands release a hormone called cortisol, our ancient fight-or-flight mechanism that helped us escape from saber-toothed tigers. Cortisol gives us that quick burst of energy, the pounding heart, the superhuman strength and heightened reflexes. But in our modern world, those saber-toothed tigers never go away and we experience chronically elevated cortisol, with a host of negative effects: high blood sugar, increased amounts of dangerous abdominal fat, high blood pressure, reduced immunity, impaired memory and the health conditions that result from these conditions.

It estimated that 90% of all visits to the doctor's office are stress-related—not illnesses that are "all in your head" or hypochondria—and we know there is a stress component to many diseases.

There are many ways to manage stress, ranging from meditation and yoga to exercise and socializing. There are also caveats: get enough sleep and avoid cigarettes and overuse of alcohol and caffeine.

Your Garden to the Rescue

There are also many food-based ways to address your stress and move into the "cool zone."

Potatoes and other starchy vegetables are good stress relievers, largely because our culture views them as comfort foods. That's because carbohydrates can actually cause changes to brain chemistry that raise levels of the feel-good brain chemical serotonin, making you feel more relaxed.

Celery can also help relieve stress-related hypertension because it relaxes muscles, including the arterial muscles that we tense up in stressful times.

The high levels of B vitamins as well as vitamins A and C in green beans affect the nervous system and help bring about a sense of calm when you are feeling jittery.

From your herb garden, **lavender** (a sprinkle of flowers in your bath water), **borage** (as a tea) and **chamomile** in any form are the quintessential stress relievers. They should be staples in your herb collection.

SUNBURN

YOUR GARDEN RX: cucumbers, eggplant, potato, tomato, chamomile

We've all been there, intentionally or not: we've been too long in the sun and find ourselves with a painful burn. When it happens only occasionally, it's a minor inconvenience. The sunburn will usually fade within days (and you most likely won't be tan underneath). You may need to avoid the friends who invariably want to slap you on the back during this time, and the outer layer of skin may peel, but in the short term, sunburn is no big deal.

In the long term, however, repeated sunburns can be a very big deal, significantly increasing your risk of skin cancers, including potentially deadly melanoma.

When you're out in the sun, wear a hat. Better yet, if you're out for more than a few minutes, put on a zinc oxide–based sunscreen, the safest kind around.

Your Garden to the Rescue

A cool **cucumber** paste will ease the pain quickly, as will pulverized **eggplant**.

Rubbing a cut potato on the burned area will ease the pain, as will a cool **chamomile** tea wash.

If you're looking for a natural sunscreen, add **tomatoes** to your diet on a regular basis. The lycopene in tomatoes gives you natural sun protection from within, but don't count on that for complete sun protection. You'll still need sunscreen (a natural one!), hat and protective clothing.

TOOTHACHE

YOUR GARDEN RX: chili peppers, oregano

Most of us get a little tooth pain from time to time—maybe from eating ice (a bad habit I have been unable to break) or tooth sensitivity to heat or cold. Tooth pain in adults, if it continues for more than a couple of days, requires dental care because it could signal a cavity, a cracked tooth, an abscess or other infection. It can even signal something serious and non–dental related; for example, it can be an uncommon signal for angina chest pain that can be a signal of heart disease.

Tooth pain in children is familiar because it signals tooth-fairy time. There is no need for dental intervention unless the tooth doesn't come out on its own.

Your Garden to the Rescue

Okay, go ahead and cringe, but a cut **hot pepper**, which will initially burn when applied to the painful area, will soon cancel out the pain signals. The pain relief will probably last two to three hours, when you can repeat the process. Hot peppers also contain salicylates—painkillers similar to aspirin.

Not yet ready to go the chili-pepper route? Try **oregano**.

Make a strong tea and swish it around in your mouth for pain relief and ammunition against infection if that is what is causing the pain.

RX from Outside Your Garden

My grandmother always kept a bottle of clove oil in her medicine cabinet, and I have fond memories of her dabbing it on my gums when my baby teeth were falling out and adult teeth coming in. The pain would vanish almost immediately.

TOXIN OVERLOAD

YOUR GARDEN RX: beets, blueberries, bok choy, broccoli, carrots, onions, apples, strawberries, milk thistle, red clover

All of us are exposed to a soup of toxins every day. Even if you are lucky enough to be able to eat a totally organic diet, you're still being bombarded by toxins all around you, ranging from polluted air to household and industrial chemicals, cosmetics and personal care products, pollutants in municipal water, cigarette smoke and off-gassing carpets and furniture in your own homes or in places you visit or work.

It is virtually impossible to avoid exposure to these toxins, but it is certainly possible to help sweep them from our systems. Since the liver is the body's primary organ of detoxification (we also detoxify through the breathing process and through our urine and sweat), look for foods that help support optimal liver function to help detoxify your body.

Your Garden to the Rescue

Beets help purify your blood and cleanse your liver with the help of a unique blend of phytochemicals.

Blueberries have a rare ability to stop toxins from crossing the blood–brain barrier and entering the fatty tissues of the brain.

Cruciferous vegetables like **bok choy, broccoli** and more contain in their health arsenal the ability to neutralize some of the pollutants in cigarette smoke and also stimulate the liver to produce the enzyme it needs for detoxification.

Beta-carotene found in **carrots, sweet potatoes** and other orange vegetables, help sweep heavy metals out of the body. The pectin in **apples** binds to the heavy metals and helps neutralize them so they can be safely eliminated from the body.

Onions, one of our superfoods, has been shown to help thin the blood, and they also cleanse it and help detoxify the respiratory tract.

Vitamin C–rich foods, like **strawberries, watermelon** and **bell peppers,** help the body produce glutathione, which supports healthy liver function and helps neutralize damage from environmental toxins.

Milk thistle has traditionally been used to protect the liver from damage from toxins, and they can also protect it from damage from certain drugs, such as acetaminophen (most commonly known as Tylenol), that can cause liver damage. Milk thistle may actually help the liver grow new cells and repair itself.

Finally, **red clover** helps the body rid itself of excess mucus and fluids. It's often prescribed by herbalists (flowers and leaves dried and used as a tea) to enhance the cleansing action of liver, kidneys and the lymphatic system.

VAGINITIS/YEAST INFECTIONS

YOUR GARDEN RX: blackberry, garlic, spinach, dried beans, oregano, chamomile, calendula

Most vaginal infections are caused by yeast overgrowth in the vagina. There is much speculation about the cause of these types of fungal infections, but it almost certainly due to dysbiosis, an imbalance of friendly and unfriendly microorganisms in the digestive tract. When the imbalance becomes extreme, *Candida albicans* yeast, which is naturally present in the digestive tract, can begin to grow out of control, eventually permeating the intestinal walls and lodging in any of a number of places in the body, including the vagina.

If you've taken antibiotics recently, that has likely contributed to the imbalance, as do taking birth control pills and excess sugar consumption (yeast literally loves to "eat" sugar). Conventional medicine sometimes treats vaginitis with antibiotics, which are useless against fungal infections.

Your Garden to the Rescue

We have an arsenal of foods and herbs that can help rein in that yeast overgrowth. **Garlic**, with its abundance of sulfur compounds, is a natural antifungal, as is **oregano**.

Blackberries, spinach and **dried beans** are good sources of the B vitamin folic acid, which may help protect you from vaginal infections.

Calendula is a natural astringent with the ability to help your body fight off all types of infections, including fungal infections. Calendula is most commonly made into a salve.

A **chamomile** tea or wash or flowers added to your bath water can ease the pain and itching associated with vaginitis.

VARICOSE VEINS

YOUR GARDEN RX: blueberries, grapes, parsley, bay leaves, cabbage

Varicose veins are ropy, enlarged veins (spider veins are smaller versions), usually in the legs, cosmetically inelegant, but most often no more than a nuisance, although sometimes they are the source of a dull ache or pain and swelling. However, varicose veins can increase your risk for more serious circulatory problems. Conventional medicine recommends compression stockings to help the veins return blood to the heart. In serious cases, various types of surgery may be considered.

Your Garden to the Rescue

Virtually all fruits and vegetables have some levels of antioxidants called flavonoids. Flavonoids like those found in **grapes** can reduce the permeability of blood vessels so the stronger blood vessels don't leak blood and fluids into the surrounding tissue. A particular flavonoid compound called rutin has been study-proven to help strengthen capillaries and improve varicose veins. You'll find rutin in **parsley, blueberries**, citrus fruits and buckwheat. **Blueberries** and **grapes** are extra helpful because they are also good sources of capillary-strengthening anthocyanins. Poultices made of **bay leaves** and/or **cabbage** warmed in olive oil have long been used as a topical remedy to reduce varicose veins and relieve swelling.

WARTS

YOUR GARDEN RX: garlic, onion, spinach, dried beans, potatoes

As many as 10% of us get these unsightly growths, which most frequently occur on hands, feet and genitals. While there is no validation for the old wives' tale that toads cause warts, it is known that warts are caused by the human papillomavirus (HPV) and they can be contagious, particularly if you are immune-compromised and you have contact with someone with genital warts.

Your Garden to the Rescue

Simply rubbing a clove of **garlic** or a sliced **onion** on an external wart can give you enough antimicrobial sulfur compounds to knock out the virus that causes warts. Some people prefer to take their garlic infused in oil or even internally. You wouldn't want to put garlic directly on genital warts or on a baby's skin, because it could be strong enough to burn. Eating **spinach, potatoes, dried beans** and other zinc-rich foods is known to help boost immune function and even specifically to help get rid of warts.

PART 3

Superfoods You Can Grow

If you've read the 101 prescriptions ailments carefully, you'll notice that certain foods appear over and over again. These foods are our superfoods, those that have the highest nutrient density and the highest variety of nutrients that are effective ways to address – and prevent—a wide variety of diseases and ailments.

There is a large body of research that shows – in my mind *proves*—that the healthiest and longest-lived humans are those who eat the most fruits and vegetables.

Superfoods multiply those health benefits untold numbers of times. I can't emphasize enough the value of superfoods. It's so great that if you eat just a serving of each of these foods every day, I can assure you that your life will be healthier and longer.

Here's my super list in the general order of their importance, in my purely subjective opinion:

1. Garlic
2. Onions
3. Spinach
4. Blueberries
5. Tomatoes
6. Beans, dried
7. Broccoli
8. Apples
9. Potatoes
10. Pumpkin/pumpkin seeds

A Rewarding Task Results in a Healthy Lifestyle

At the beginning of this book, I set out to give you the secrets of health and long life with foods you can grow or buy close to home. I hope you've gained some valuable insight into the myriad of ways the foods you eat—and the foods you grow right in your own backyard or on your own deck or windowsill—will not only keep you healthy, but also address your health complaints.

Whether you're treating insect bites, sunburn and canker sores or cancer, heart disease, diabetes and everything in between, the foods you eat are the foundation of your health and your recovery.

Yes, supplements can be helpful. Yes, sometimes you need medical attention and all the power that modern medicine and prescription drugs can offer. I always remember Dr. Andrew Weil's comment: "If I'm in a car accident, don't take me to an herbalist!" Still, the foods you eat and the nutritional status you've established will unquestionably have great influence on the outcome of your health challenges.

For most of us, most of the time, the foods we can grow in our own gardens or buy close to where they were grown are our greatest allies in wellness, our most powerful preventive tools, our most potent curatives and the source of great joy.

Hopefully, armed with helpful info, you're inspired to start a garden or get out into your already-established garden, feel the sun on your shoulders and savor the freshest food on earth. As I write this, I am snacking on a dozen cherry tomatoes picked from my garden ten minutes ago. What a gift!

I'd like to hear your health and gardening experiences. Please visit my website, www.kathleenbarnes.com, to offer comments and complaints, or e-mail me directly at kathleen@kathleenbarnes.com. You find me on Facebook at: www.facebook.com/kathleen.barnes.nc and on Twitter @kathleensbarnes.

Resources

Websites

Kathleen Barnes: *www.kathleenbarnes.com*

WebMd: *www.webmd.com*

Natural Cures: *www.naturalcures.com*

The Cancer Cure Foundation: *www.cancure.org*

Natural Health News: *www.naturalnews.com*

Dr. Hyla Cass: *www.cassmd.com*

Pharmacist Suzy Cohen: *www.dearpharmacist.com*

Dr. James Duke: *www.greenpharmacy.com*

Chris Kilham, The Medicine Hunter: *www.medicinehunter.com*

Dr. Joe Mercola: *www.mercola.com*

Dr. Ray Sahelian: *www.raysahelian.com*

Dr. Jacob Teitelbaum: *www.endfatigue.com*

Dr. Andrew Weil: *www.drweil.com*

Gardens Alive! (source for nontoxic pesticides, herbicides, and fertilizers and great resource for pest control and disease identification information): *www.gardensalive.com*

Spray-N-Grow natural fertilizers: *www.spray-n-grow.com*

About the Author

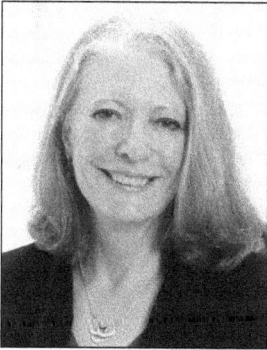

Kathleen Barnes is an ardent advocate of natural health and an equally avid gardener. Her career as a journalist and writer has spanned more than four decades, including years as an international correspondent for ABC and CNN during historic transitions in the Philippines and South Africa. In recent years, she has turned her writing to natural health and sustainable living, writing and editing 20 books.

She has written extensively for national and international publications, including more than six years as the weekly natural health columnist for *Woman's World* magazine.

Kathleen lives in the Blue Ridge Mountains of western North Carolina with her husband, Joe, and an ever-changing extended family of horses, dogs, cats and the occasional pond frog.

Kathleen Barnes' other books include:

The Calcium Lie 2: What Your Doctor Still Doesn't Know with Dr. Robert Thompson (Take Charge Books, 2013)

10 Best Ways to Mange Stress (Take Charge Books, 2013)

Eight Weeks to Vibrant Health: A Take Charge Plan for Women with Dr. Hyla Cass. (Take Charge Books, 2008 second edition, first edition McGraw-Hill).

The Calcium Lie: What Your Doctor Doesn't Know Might Kill You with Dr. Robert Thompson. (Take Charge Books, 2008).

The Secret of Health: Breast Wisdom with Dr. Ben Johnson. (Morgan James Publishing 2007).

User's Guide to Thyroid Disorders. (Basic Health Publications, 2006).

User's Guide to Natural Hormone Replacement. (Basic Health Publications, 2006).

Arthritis and Joint Health. (Woodland Publishing, 2005).

www.ingramcontent.com/pod-product-compliance
Lightning Source LLC
Chambersburg PA
CBHW060902280326

41934CB00007B/1154